DHEA
The Ultimate Rejuvenating Hormone

DHEA
The Ultimate Rejuvenating Hormone

Hasnain Walji, Ph.D.

HOHM PRESS
Prescott, Arizona

HOHM PRESS
PO Box 2501
Prescott, AZ 86302
520-778-9189

http://www.booknotes.com/hohm/

Cover: Kim Johansen, Black Dog Design
Layout: AV Communications, Mesa, AZ.

Walji, Hasnain.
    DHEA : the ultimate rejuvenating hormone / Hasnain Walji.
    p.   cm.
    Includes bibliographical references and index.
    ISBN 0-934252-70-X
    1. Dehydroepiandrosterone—Therapeutic use.
    2. Dehydroepiandrosterone—Physiological effect.   I. Title.
    RM296.5.D45W35   1996
    615'.364—dc21   96-43991
                                                        CIP

ISBN: 0-934252-70-X

Disclaimer: No information in this book is intended to be a replacement for medical advice. Any person with a condition requiring medical attention should consult a qualified health professional.

Dedication

Whilst the book may assist the victim of disease,
I dedicate it to the seekers of health.

Acknowledgments

I would like to express my gratitude to my editor Regina Sara Ryan at Hohm Press for her painstaking review of the manuscript and offering many pertinent suggestions and to David Ponsonby without whose contribution, in research and subediting, it would not have been possible to write this book.

Last but not least, I wish to thank my wife Latifa whose gentle care and concern enabled me to complete this book.

Contents

Preface

"Life begins at forty," we say in a half-hearted attempt to bolster self-confidence (either our own or someone else's), but unconvincingly. Deep down, we have been socialized to think: "I am over the hill now." But, while "the exception proves the rule" haven't we all wondered why some 50 year-olds look and act a decade younger, while others look 65 — or older?

While there is more to aging than simply the passage of time, youth does tend to benefit from every body system operating at closer to peak efficiency. As we get older, we become increasingly prone to degenerative diseases. The same flu which kept us home from work for a few days can now prove to be a fatal disease. Instead of a six week convalescence for a broken bone, this condition in an elderly person may prove to be terminal. In the later stage of life, it becomes critical to ensure that the body is operating at its optimum level.

The relationship between aging and degeneration is not as inevitable as we have accepted. Senility and death at around 70 is not a foregone conclusion — we have some control over the rate at which we age. The key to how we feel, think and look is related to the optimum functioning of our body systems. While it is true that we cannot control the passage of time, we do influence the ravages of time by our lifestyle and diet. In particular, as we spend more time in our loungers, we hasten the day when we cannot get up and walk around. If we continue to overeat, especially if we have a reduced level of activity, the "middle-age spread" is going to increase. Over the long-term, every system is damaged: the blood doesn't flow, the oxygen doesn't reach the cells, the cells don't function properly, the food doesn't digest well, etc.

In terms of freedom from disease, or wellness as distinct from illness, a functional immune system will sustain optimum health but a depressed immune system will be over-powered by every disease-causing organism, radiation treatment or chemical onslaught.

Longevity with health and vitality are closely related to the secretion of hormones. Medical prescriptions support this: estrogen replacement therapy has been a boon to many postmenopausal women and now testosterone patches may provide similar benefits to "andropausal" men. However, it is not the intention of the author to promote prescription drugs as a means of preserving youthfulness. These are last-minute interventions following a long process of decline. Hormonal replacement therapy represents, for the most part, symptomatic relief — it does not alter the underlying causes. Twentieth century environmental factors and an imbalanced diet have taken their toll on our health and well being.

Deliberate action is called for to avoid environmental pollution and to select clean water and non-toxic foods, thereby enabling the body to fulfill its natural course, which seems to be a vigorous life beyond the century mark, as demonstrated by several well-publicized (but isolated) populations, like the Hunzas.

Scientific research abounds with studies confirming that the human body functions best when supplemented with essential nutrients in correct amounts (otherwise we suffer from "Too much of a good thing"!). The nutrition connection, therefore, has to be one of the more important links in the chain. Maintaining good health requires a concerted effort to combat the destructive barrage which assaults the body day after day, year after year.

The most publicized dysfunction is probably oxidation, i.e., the production of free radicals. Thus, the contemporary interest in antioxidants, i.e., nutrients which counter the free radicals and support the oxidative processes. Antioxidant vitamins (such as vitamins A, C and E) and minerals (such as selenium) have been joined by hormones like melatonin which benefit oxidation and thereby counter the degenerative processes associated with aging. Depending upon one's viewpoint, the degenerative processes are not so much a consequence of the accumulated years but the accumulation of free radicals, or the deterioration of the oxidative processes.

Now another hormone, DHEA, is fast achieving prominence in that arsenal of forces to counteract the attack of free radicals and other degenerative processes. In the ever elusive quest for the elixir of youth, the so called "baby boomers" seem to have found the answer in this hormone. This book is an attempt to help the reader through the maze of contradictions regarding DHEA.

As the claims and counterclaims, by vested interests, surface on the efficacy (short- and long-term) of DHEA, we must not lose sight of the fallacy of relying on magic pills to maintain optimum health and attain longevity. We should not fall into the torturous trap of medicalization —dependency on modern medical intervention; of allowing ourselves to become broken down before seeking a quick fix. We must take full responsibility for our own health. The toxic load in the modern world is, however, too great. To rely solely upon organic foods is not enough. Supplementation with selected nutrients is now essential.

One of the clearest biomarkers during the aging process is the level of DHEA circulating in the blood. Hence, we may have reached the point at which even minerals and vitamins are no longer adequate for total health, and hormones must be added to the list. For some people, this is too close to the medical paradigm for comfort, even via herbal sources. This group may signpost the way for the rest of us into the realm of the mind-body relationship. Mind and body are aspects of the human whole; interrelated and indivisible from each other. When all is said and done, you are *"only as old as you feel."*

Hasnain Walji, Ph.D.
September 1996

A Note Concerning the Legal Status of DHEA

The market position of DHEA has also remained confusing, so that some people may still think that it is available only by prescription. DHEA, like vitamin C or any other nutrient, is available on prescription but not exclusively so. It is a nutritional supplement available over-the-counter, or via mail order. However, only a physician can order the blood tests to determine blood levels of natural DHEA upon which basis a therapeutic protocol should be founded. Current research involves multiple sclerosis and lupus, for example. Such conditions are normally under the care of a physician, anyway. DHEA nutritional supplementation applies more to a broad-spectrum anti-aging strategy in the absence of chronic disease. If you are under the care of a physician, it is always prudent to mention your intended nutritional supplementation program in case of any potential for negative interactions.

1

Did You Know

WHAT DO HEALTH CONDITIONS as diverse as aging, AIDS, cancer, heart disease, diabetes, obesity and osteoporosis all have in common? Would it surprise you to know that there is a growing body of research which suggests that each of these conditions is marked by a deficiency, or low blood levels, of a substance called *dehydroepiandrosterone,* (pronounced dee-hi-dro-epp-ee-ann-dro-stehr-own) — DHEA for short — that is produced by the adrenal glands but is not just another hormone? Dr. William Regelson, a noted researcher specializing in aging, or more accurately anti-aging, calls DHEA the "mother hormone" because the body is able to convert it into major hormones such as estrogen, testosterone and adrenaline, as needed.

Hormones are chemical substances produced by various glands or organs. They are a part of the complex regulatory processes in our bodies. Usually we associate hormones with negative images of unwanted hair, pimples and obesity. This is because we only tend to be told about hormones when there are imbalances in the body. Nothing could be further from the truth. Hormones have a powerful impact on every cell!

A hormone that has attracted considerable publicity recently is melatonin. The role melatonin played in the functioning of the body was, until recently, a mystery. In 1987, B. R. Grad and Dr. Roman Rozencwaig were among the first to postulate a theory that aging was a syndrome of melatonin deficiency, which itself resulted from the gradual failure of the pineal gland. Since then the impact of melatonin deficiency has been extensively researched and, to date, over 4,500 scientific papers have been published on the multifarious implications of melatonin. It is now widely believed that melatonin may have a major role to play in the management of sleep disorders, jet lag and numerous auto-immune diseases, in addition to its ability to retard the aging process.

In the same manner, though known to scientists for over half a century, DHEA received little attention until recently. Now, there is a growing body of research that suggests that DHEA has many more important functions in the body than previously believed. Indeed, research which is now emerging suggests that DHEA may well be the most critical substance in the body; one that determines the very levels of health and disease.

WHERE DOES DHEA COME FROM?

Made in the body from cholesterol, the apparent paradox is that often DHEA levels decline with age while cholesterol levels rise. DHEA is a steroid like the other steroid hormones — estrogen, progesterone and testosterone. However, DHEA is produced in far greater quantities than any other hormone produced by the adrenal glands. Until quite recently it was not known why the adrenal glands made DHEA and what DHEA's function was. What scientists knew was that DHEA could be converted into other hormones including estrogen and testosterone. Science called DHEA a buffer hormone, meaning a reservoir from which the body could produce other hormones. With greater focus on DHEA, it now appears that this remarkable hormone has very important functions of its own and is emerging as one of the most effective substances against the ravages of twentieth century living.

This chapter will provide an overview of significant highlights from some of the latest research on DHEA. This more complete picture of DHEA shows it emerging as one of the most potent health-giving substances. In subsequent chapters we will look at these significant highlights in more detail.

THE ANTI-AGING HORMONE

The link between aging and certain hormones is exciting scientists all over the world. Now DHEA has joined the ranks of hormones like estrogen and melatonin, and seems poised to be touted as another "miracle drug" by the media. Indeed, the CBS news magazine *Eye to Eye* set the ball rolling in June 1995, followed by articles in *The New York Times* and the *Washington Post*.

Such high-profile coverage can be a two-edged sword. While it introduces the cutting edge (pun intentional) of nutritional therapy, it inevitably risks the ire of the drug barons and the pharmaceutical lobby who stand to miss out on millions of dollars of potential income because natural substances, like DHEA, cannot be patented. Therefore it is highly unlikely that the drug barons will fund any research. It does not make commercial sense to invest millions without any protection for the product being developed. In the meantime, the U.S. Food and Drug Administration (FDA) continues to issue obtuse statements, saying that they have had few diverse reaction reports on the drug, and that the risks from long-term use are unknown. While the U.S. Drug Enforcement Administration has tentatively decided not to classify DHEA as a scheduled drug.

Considering that DHEA is the only hormone that progressively diminishes in the body after ages 20-25, its presence (or lack of presence) is considered to be a reliable marker of aging. The body is apparently programmed to reduce the natural production of DHEA, thus giving way to the process of aging. Indeed, it is now becoming evident that DHEA is much more than a reservoir or precursor hormone that the body can draw upon to synthesize other hormones.

There is a new view that cells in the human body contain specific DHEA receptors whose only function is to bind DHEA. In simple terms, this means that DHEA has a direct influence on cellular activity and stability, both of which have a major impact upon the rate at which we age.

Numerous studies show that when DHEA was fed to mice it increased their life expectancy by a third. The treated mice seemed younger and had a lower incidence of the typical diseases of aging. DHEA reduced the risk of breast, colon and lung cancer in mice. According to biochemist Dr. Norman Applezweig, DHEA "de-excites" the body's processes and some of the diseases of aging caused by runaway production of nucleic acids, fats and hormones. DHEA regulates their production and thereby slows down aging.

It is this age-slowing aspect of the hormone that is the culmination of many of the specific conditions discussed above. In this era of "baby boomers," any substance that retards the aging process will inevitably prove popular. DHEA appears to bear all the hallmarks of "The Wonder Substance" that can offer hope to millions in their quest for an elixir of youth. Is such a thing possible? The sixty-four-thousand-dollar question is: If DHEA levels are a measure of our youth, is it possible to retain youth and vigor by increasing these levels? This discussion will be developed fully in the later chapters.

Further, it is interesting to follow the work of two researchers who are at opposite ends of the debate on the long-term impact of DHEA. In his article, "Forever Young" (Sept/Oct issue of *Science*, published by The New York Academy of Sciences), Burkhard Bilger reports on the conference on DHEA and aging hosted by the Academy. In the article he quotes John Nestler (whose own research has shown that high doses of DHEA can lower cholesterol levels) as saying: "I think that they are jumping the gun. People said that the human growth hormone was great stuff at first too, but now we are seeing significant side effects...bloating, carpal tunnel syndrome. The same thing could happen with DHEA."

In stark contrast, William Regelson, who is described as "an old hand at rabble-rousing for research on aging," is quoted in the same article to say: "I respect John Nestler ... He is a top-flight scientist. But the guy is forty-two years old! ... He can afford to be conservative. I'll be seventy on July 12. (He looks twenty years younger.) It's like somebody out there has a contract out there to kill me. I do not want to wait twenty or thirty years. I want it now!"

Such is the passion of the debate even among experts and leading authorities on DHEA. Are there good reasons to think that taking a DHEA supplement adds years to your life and life to your years? In the chapters to follow we shall demystify all the issues to help you make an informed decision on whether to take DHEA now or wait twenty or thirty years, or ignore it altogether as the proverbial "hype."

Do Low DHEA Levels Double the Risk of AIDS ?

In an article in *The Journal of Infectious Diseases* (November, 1991) researcher William Regelson reported that people with the HIV virus do not seem to develop full-blown AIDS until their body's output of DHEA falls. He also found that HIV-positive men with low DHEA levels had double the risk of getting full-blown AIDS compared to those with normal DHEA levels.

Can Low DHEA Levels Contribute to Breast Cancer?

As early as 1962, researchers in England (Bulbrook, 1962, 1971) reported that DHEA was abnormally low in women who developed breast cancer. In a study on 5,000 apparently healthy women, it was found that all twenty-seven of the women who developed and died of breast cancer had blood levels of DHEA less than 10% of the norm for their age group. Further, that these women had subnormal DHEA levels up to nine years before their cancer was diagnosed. The key question, which we will try to answer in this book, is: If low DHEA levels contributed to breast cancer might the opposite be true? Namely, whether taking

DHEA supplements and restoring youthful levels would prevent or reverse the disease process.

Can Administering DHEA Really Lower the Incidence of Heart Disease?

According to a study published in the *New England Journal of Medicine* (1986), Elizabeth Barrett-Connor, M.D., at the University of California School of Medicine in San Diego, observed DHEA levels in 242 men, ages 50-79, for twelve years. In men with a history of heart disease DHEA levels were significantly lower than men with no history of heart disease. Further, Barrett-Connor and other researchers concluded that even in people without heart disease, DHEA seems to protect against early death. Can administering DHEA really lower the incidence of heart disease? A 1988 study, at John Hopkins Medical Institute, used DHEA on rabbits with severe arteriosclerosis. The result was an almost 50% reduction in plaque size.

What Role Does DHEA Play in Immune Enhancement?

DHEA has been shown to confer a special protection against viral infections. *The Harvard Health Letter*, July 1994, contained an article entitled, "DHEA Gets Respect." It was reported that DHEA added to vaccines helped older mice develop the same vigorous antibodies as young mice. This study is of particular interest. If such a reaction could be replicated in humans it would have exciting possibilities in delaying the onset of disease in the elderly (preferably until after death; or in the spirit of Dr. Russell Reiter, a prominent scientist, people will die *young* at an advanced age). Richard Hodes, the director of the National Institute of Aging, observes that these implications are "extremely interesting and potentially important."

What Impact on Memory?

DHEA has been shown to improve memory in aging mice, according to Dr. Robert Atkins (*Health Revelation*, January 1994). Animal experiments have demonstrated that even minimal amounts lessen amnesia and promote long-term memory. In human subjects, research showed that blood levels of DHEA in a group of Alzheimer's patients were 48% lower than in the control group.

An interesting example is cited by Dr. Kenneth Bonnet, a research scientist in the Department of Psychiatry at New York University School of Medicine. Within one week of receiving low doses of DHEA, a forty-seven-year-old woman (with lifelong multiple learning disabilities and low memory retention) showed an improvement in recall ability. Upon increasing the dosage, tests confirmed further improvements.

Does DHEA Lower Body Weight Regardless of Caloric Intake ?

Arthur Schwartz, the researcher at Temple University in Philadelphia who found that DHEA blocks a fat-producing enzyme (G6PD), says that, "DHEA is a very effective anti-obesity agent." Animal studies suggest that DHEA may be effective in treating obesity. In a strain of mice with a predisposition to obesity, administering 500 mg. per kilo of body weight prevented the development of obesity. What is also important is that since no loss of appetite was noted, this indicates that the effect of DHEA was to speed up metabolism. Calories consumed were simply converted to heat rather than stored as fat. At the same time, DHEA helps the body to produce lean muscle tissue (Yen, 1977). Can such effects be replicated in humans? What impact would it have on athletic training and sports nutrition? These aspects are attracting wide attention. "One of the reasons for the great interest in DHEA is its apparent ability to lower body weight regardless of caloric intake," says biochemist Dr. Neecie Moore. The impact of this research could be monumental in weight loss methods.

Natural or Synthetic?

Synthetic DHEA is being tested in laboratory conditions with some effective results. But as with all synthetic drugs, the question is always, could synthetic DHEA have unwanted side effects? Some fifty years ago, scientists discovered that a rare Mexican plant called *Dioscorea*, often called the Mexican yam, contained the basic DHEA compound in the precursor form which our bodies can then use to manufacture DHEA. Although science has known about *Dioscorea* for half a century, the significance of it has been recognized only during the past decade or so, following the findings on the importance of DHEA. However, there are some who believe that the yam source may not really be able to provide DHEA in the required quantities.

Miracle or a Drug?

While the medical establishment drags its feet in endorsing the benefits of DHEA despite thousands of studies, some progressive physicians, like Dr. Julian Whitaker, M.D., feel more confident. In his newsletter, *Health & Healing,* Whitaker writes: "... the number of areas in which supplemental DHEA is helpful is almost alarming, because it covers such a broad range." Among other health professionals who endorse natural nutrition as preventive to disease, nutritionist Dr. Richard Passwater says succinctly: "Anybody over 25 should be supplementing their diet with DHEA."

DHEA is neither a miracle nor a *drug,* in the strict sense of the word; it is naturally present in the human body. DHEA levels are abundant in both men and women until about twenty years of age. Up to the early thirties, we typically produce about 30 mg. per day of DHEA. As we grow older our levels decrease, dwindling to under 5 mg. per day in our sixties. There are hardly any traces of the hormone in the body at the time of death.

So, even those who are normally skeptical about any cure-all are beginning to acknowledge the comprehensive impact of DHEA. The expanding research on DHEA means that orthodox healthcare professionals can no longer ignore or deny it. In later chapters we will delve into greater detail on every aspect of all the current research on the management of degenerative diseases of twentieth-century Western civilization, and investigate the process of aging which seems to have become a particular obsession of our youth dominated culture.

2

A Measure of Youth

THE CONNECTION BETWEEN
AGING AND DHEA LEVELS

WHY WE AGE, OR rather *how* the process starts, is a matter of some conjecture. There seem to be three main theories that have been offered so far. Let us look at each of these in turn.

1. The Cell-Related Theory of Aging

This theory has to do with how well our cells function. It has been suggested that, at some stage in our lives, errors and changes in our DNA cause mutation or damage to our cells and, consequently, substandard and insufficient protein is produced, the result of which is that our bodies cannot adequately repair and maintain themselves. Thus the system starts to break down. A linked idea is that our cells are pre-programmed by our DNA to age, in the same way that they are programmed to grow and develop.

Free radicals enter into this cell-related theory. They are credited with going on the rampage and damaging the DNA or else causing the cells to malfunction so that their ability to detoxify themselves and perform their other functions is impaired and, again, the system breaks down. Free radicals are implicated in such symptoms of aging as wrinkles, together with faulty enzyme activity and sugar-related alterations. They can cause cross-linking between cells, which affects collagen, the "glue" that holds us all together.

2. The Organ-Related Theory of Aging

This next theory proposes that, as the non-replaceable parts of our bodies wear out, we simply function steadily less well until we stop functioning altogether. There may also be the added effect of the build-up of toxins; we become increasingly unable to get rid of toxins because of organ deterioration.

Another explanation that fits within the organ-related theory of aging is that aging is the consequence of hormonal disturbances or changes in the functioning of the immune system.

3. Integrated Theory of Aging

The third theory is really a synthesis of these first two and is sometimes called the integrated theory of aging. It recognizes that there is an underlying, genetically pre-programmed duration of life that is then influenced for better or worse at the cellular level by other factors, such as toxicity, stress, nutritional deficiencies, energy, infections and so on. Organ dysfunction may result, and eventually the body can no longer cope. It is the outside factors that need to be tackled if we want to ensure a healthy old age and live in that happy state for as long as we can. (One hundred twenty years is one estimate of our potential life expectancy!)

WHERE DO THESE THEORIES LEAVE US?

All three of these theories beg the question, but what actually starts the whole aging process off?

Some scientists believe that the signals to start aging (which are contained in our DNA) are switched on once a particular level of toxicity and inefficiency is reached. The alterations that then take place are discussed in Leon Chaitow's book *Natural Life Extension* (London: Thorsons, 1992). These alterations include:

- The process whereby the cross-linkage of proteins and fats is disrupted, leading to a build-up of age pigments (lipofuscin).
- Digestive enzymes deteriorate and lose their functional ability and contribute weakly to the immune system.
- Brain tissue appears to be tangled, like an old ball of string, which is best known in the neurodegenerative disease called Alzheimer's.

Research has shown that where cells are able to detoxify themselves efficiently and the repair of DNA is at its optimum, there is a coincidentally longer life span. Scientists now suggest that DHEA appears to be necessary for duplication of DNA.

APPROACHES TO LONGER LIFE

There have been three main approaches to achieving a longer life, all of which are supported by laboratory evidence rather than by direct experimentation on humans, although population studies have tended to bear out the conclusions of the animal studies. These approaches are:

- calorie restriction
- antioxidant nutrition to counteract free radicals
- the use of amino acids to trigger growth hormone production.

Let us now look at each of these ideas in more detail.

Dietary Restriction

It seems from animal studies that modifications and restrictions made to diet result in far fewer illnesses — including cardiovascular disease, cancer, diabetes, arthritis and dementia, among others — than would otherwise be the case. If such diseases or conditions do occur, they do so much later in the life of the animal. "Dietary restriction" means a diet containing all the necessary nutrients but with a much lower calorie content than the norm.

Built in to dietary restriction are periods of fasting. Fasting has been shown to reduce the body's basic metabolic rate (BMR), the rate at which it burns "fuel" for energy production. This makes our energy consumption more efficient and increases life span. Fasting also results in certain hormonal changes, particularly an increase in production of growth hormone by the pituitary gland. Diseases can be dealt with through fasting, too, including diabetes, gangrene, heart disease, pancreatitis, rheumatoid arthritis, food allergy and varicose ulcers, to name but a few.

What seems to happen during dietary restriction is that lipofuscin (the age pigment) is reduced, which in turn slows down the rate of aging. The number of free radicals is reduced too, as the body becomes more efficient at burning its fuel, and the core body temperature is lowered. Protein synthesis changes, and self-repair is enhanced.

Antioxidant Nutrition

There is evidence both for and against the free-radical theory of aging. One argument *against* it is that the process of aging seems to fit a recognized pattern, whereas free-radical damage is haphazard. Earlier, it was suggested that aging may depend on the interplay between genetic programming and levels of damage and toxicity. There is, of course, the increasingly accepted view that free-radical damage is the cause of a large number of degenerative diseases, including heart disease, cancer, cataracts and Alzheimer's disease. Whether or not a reduction in the number of free radicals actually prolongs life or simply improves the quality of life in the elderly, it is obvious that we should do all we can to reduce the burden free radicals place on our bodies.

The best way of going about this — apart from, perhaps, dietary restriction — is to consume foods rich in antioxidants and, possibly, to take antioxidant supplements.

Use of Amino Acids

Interest in supplementation with the amino acids *arginine* and *ornithine* so as to stimulate the pituitary gland into making more growth hormone was prevalent in the early 1980s. This hormone is responsible for growth and repair and has been shown to benefit the immune system. It can help to decrease fatty tissue, increase lean body mass, increase the density of bone and thicken the skin. But, by the time we reach sixty, many of us have none of this hormone present.

Growth hormone production is not only stimulated by amino acids, however. Other factors that promote it are peak level exercise, trauma, fasting and sleep.

The question remains: If DHEA levels are a measure of our youth is it possible to retain youth and vigor by increasing these levels? The generation of post Second World War "baby boomers" is now fifty years of age and possesses a collective will to ignore the current lifespan of seventy-six years and its attendant diseases (notably physical infirmity and mental incapacity). DHEA seems to have every appearance of being an answer to their prayers.

First, the older you are the less DHEA you have. In other words, DHEA levels decline in a direct relationship with age. In terms of a graph this means that there is a straight, downward slope from no later than thirty years of age which falls to zero and cuts across the age axis at the point of death.

Second, when there is a disease state, DHEA levels typically measure below this line (even relative to non-diseased persons of the same age and gender). This may be interpreted in several ways.

- Perhaps an acceleration of the age-related decline in DHEA lowers resistance to disease?
- Or a disease state (e.g., adrenal dysfunction) brings about the fall in DHEA levels.
- Alternatively, falling DHEA levels speed up the entire aging process.
- And, finally, there is some interconnected triangular relationship, with each apex: DHEA, aging and disease, intricately and inextricably linked to the next.

Third, and this may be the good news, the paradox contained in the second point may remain moot if DHEA levels can be improved, especially over the long-term. This constitutes the topic of a later chapter, but quite obviously depends upon whether one is dealing from the vantage point of a healthy thirty year old, or an elderly person suffering the ravages of disease.

It may prove best to take the preventive medicine approach and seek to maintain the DHEA levels of a healthy thirty year old as long as possible. At the very least, the rates of decline should be reduced, with respect to all three factors: DHEA levels should stay at levels consistent with youthful health and vigor; the effects of aging should be reduced; and diseases, so often confused as inevitable consequences of aging, should be more distinct and strike less often, or with reduced severity.

However, if someone is already middle-aged or elderly, even in the absence of disease, this approach would be somewhat negated. Can the decline be reversed and youthful levels restored to any meaningful degree?

Finally, in cases of chronic, incurable disease, like Alzheimer's, is there any benefit to be gained from the administration of DHEA? Without the prospect of a cure, would DHEA merely prolong the agony?

The scientific community, as a whole, must wait until the research studies are completed before reaching a conclusion about the efficacy of DHEA, like any other substance. Since many of these studies have not even begun, the results won't be in for decades. They caution us to hasten slowly. Most of us feel the urgent need to make a decision, now. The older we are, the more likely it is that we will echo the sentiment of Dr. Regelson: "We want it now!"

We may not know quite what we do want, except that we do want to be able to do *something*, rather than wait and see what the ravages of time will do to us personally and to our friends and loved ones.

At the most basic level, the risk-benefit debate boils down to the distinct possibility of added vitality and increased resistance to disease from a natural hormone at biological levels, against the certain knowledge (as Keynes phrased it) that: "... in the long run we are all dead."

While many studies have yet to be done, a number of reports are already available in prestigious medical journals, and not all of them benefited rodents! As is so often the case, the first hint that DHEA provided a fountain of youth, at least to mice, came as an incidental finding during a cancer experiment.

At the Fels Institute of Temple University, Dr. Arthur Schwartz fed DHEA to a special breed of Avy'a mice who are vulnerable to breast cancer formation. The results, published in

Cancer Research (1979) showed that the mice remained cancer-free, which is remarkable enough in itself, but Dr. Schwartz also noted that their lifespan increased 50%: "Old mice regained youthful vigor and their coats resumed their former sleek and glossy texture."

Actually, Dr. Regelson conducted some experiments with mice which led to his own use of DHEA. In this case, the transfer of information from laboratory experiments to human usage does not seem so ridiculous, or as gigantic, as in some other instances. The mice maintained their youthful hair color, texture and lean body mass. Of course, in the well-known case of former President Ronald Reagan, his youthful appearance has not prevented the onset of Alzheimer's disease.

Dr. Elizabeth Barrett-Connor, M.D., from the Department of Community and Family Medicine at the University of California School of Medicine in San Diego, has been at the forefront of this work. She followed a group of 242 men, aged between 50 and 79, for twelve years, monitoring their levels of DHEA sulfate (DHEA-S). The results, published in the *New England Journal of Medicine* (1986), showed that men with DHEA-S levels 100 micrograms per deciliter higher than others, enjoyed 48% less cardiovascular disease and 36% reduced mortality from any cause. DHEA-S provided protection against premature death.

Dr. Barrett-Connor has not been comfortable with the credit for this interest in DHEA. She feels that those physicians who have recommended this substance to their patients are acting hastily. A follow-up experiment failed to provide the startling results of the original study, lowering the risk of heart disease by just 20%.

More recently, the most celebrated studies have been conducted by Dr. Samuel Yen, professor of Reproductive Medicine at the University of California School of Medicine, also in San Diego. One 1990 study was published in the *Journal of Clinical Endocrinology and Metabolism* (1994). In the standard, double-blind, placebo-controlled format, thirteen men and seventeen women took 50 mg. of DHEA orally, at bedtime. Fully 67% of the men and 84% of the women reported an increased sense of well-being while taking the supplement. For comparison, less than 10% reported such an improvement while on the placebo. Naturally, at the time of completing the questionnaires, neither the patients, nor the doctors, knew who was taking the DHEA or the inert substance.

Dr. Yen conducted a similar trial in 1993, which he reported to the 1995 New York Academy of Sciences meeting on DHEA and aging. This time the dose was 100 mg. Within two weeks, DHEA blood levels were restored to levels found in young adults. The levels have been sustained over the period of this and other studies, at least three months. The groups in this trial were even smaller (eight men and eight women) than in the 1990 study, although Dr. Yen has announced plans for an international collaboration with French researchers in order to confirm that the changes hold true for everybody and over the long term. Dr. Yen's preliminary conclusion is that: "DHEA replacement may, at a future date, be applicable for clinical use in the aging population."

As far as large numbers of men (including some who are not so old) are concerned, a reversal of the aging process need only provide a restoration of their erectile function to claim their unswerving allegiance to the therapy. Eventual liver failure would be a better fate than sexual dysfunction. A similar dilemma has existed for many athletes: whether to take anabolic steroids in order to win a gold medal, or have a career in the NFL, at the cost of liver disease. The dining room conversation for the older generation attending the N.Y. Academy of Sciences conference in 1995 included boasts of regained potency.

For many people, that future is now! However, returning to the evidence from rodents, the best way to delay aging in a mouse is to underfeed it. Without a clear understanding of the way in which DHEA works, we could be stumbling up the wrong "garden path." DHEA could be simply suppressing our appetite. Of course, this would be a wonderful thing for the *growing* numbers of Americans fighting problems with morbid obesity and its attendant diseases, notably diabetes, which is another chapter in our story about DHEA.

3

The Smart Hormone: The Connection Between the Brain and DHEA

DR. ERIC BRAVERMAN (1995) HAS noted that brain tissue naturally contains 6.5 times more DHEA than is found in other tissues. Another researcher, James M. Howard (1995), states that the human brain's increased ability to capture DHEA is responsible for the brain's phenomenal growth at the expense of other organs. As the brain finishes growth and development, DHEA levels increase. Afterwards, during the second and third decades of life, the extra DHEA is used for higher functioning, including decision-making and reproductive drives. This makes it one of the so-called "Smart Drugs."

Viewed from the other end of the continuum, the linear relationship between DHEA and age is verifiable as a component in senile dementia, notably Alzheimer's disease, during the sixth and seventh decades of life.

Furthermore, Howard has developed these facts into an elaborate theory of human evolution in which DHEA is intricately connected to brain size and function. This provides a chemical explanation of why human beings are so superior to their nearest relatives, apes, when their basic make-up (written in the form of DNA) differs by only 1.2 per cent.

Howard has reviewed the literature concerning three disorders, at different stages of life, which serve to demonstrate his underlying hypothesis: SIDS, Alzheimer's disease and schizophrenia.

- *SIDS* (Sudden Infant Death Syndrome ; "Cot death," or "Crib death")
  Children who succumb to SIDS (they basically stop breathing) tend to have a greater brain weight. This reduces the available DHEA to undermine the brain stem, which controls the heart and breathing. At the same time, low DHEA may correlate with excess melatonin, such that there is lower consciousness during the wake cycle and deeper sleep.

- *Alzheimer's Disease*
  DHEA naturally declines with advancing age, as the incidence of neurodegenerative diseases increases. The incidence of Alzheimer's disease (AD) at 65 years of age is around 3 per cent, reaching 19 per cent by age 84 and a staggering 47 per cent in those over 85.

  This is more than a mathematical correlation. Sunderland has reported levels of DHEA in AD patients to be half that of age-matched controls, who were, themselves, 50 percent lower than youthful controls. Thus, AD patients have barely one quarter of their peak levels of DHEA.

Because REM (rapid eye movement) sleep has been implicated in memory storage, a study by Friess undertook spectral analysis of selected EEG (electroencephalograph, i.e., brain waves) bands. The print-out revealed significantly enhanced EEG activity in the *sigma* frequency range during REM sleep in the first two hour sleep period after DHEA administration. This suggests the potential clinical usefulness of DHEA in age-related dementia.

- *Schizophrenia*
  Schizophrenics are reported in the medical literature to exhibit significantly reduced levels of DHEA. They also have low melatonin. This conforms to the classic "burn-out" image of "burning the candle at both ends." Both wake and sleep cycles are impaired, which produces a vicious cycle, each further undermining the other.

Consequently, there are a large number of researchers conducting experiments with laboratory animals, as well as human trials with the intention of improving our understanding of the mechanisms involved in brain development, functioning and disorders.

Also, of course, there is question about the extension of the principle that if a substance can restore brain function can it also enhance it in normal people? DHEA is being looked at and experimented with as a so-called "Smart Food."

Dr. Ward Dean is the "guru" of this movement, providing the standard text, *Smart Drugs and Nutrients*. He states that: "DHEA protects brain cells from Alzheimer's disease and other senility-associated degenerative conditions. Nerve degeneration occurs most readily under low DHEA conditions." There is quite a lot of substantiation for Dean's views in the scientific literature.

SMART MICE

Using a (T-shaped) maze test, mice receiving DHEA demonstrated memory enhancement. Basically, the mice were trained to enter a particular section of the maze, receiving a shock if they dallied in the wrong portion. Once they had learned which section to go to five out of every six times, they would be "graduated." Upon being returned to the maze, a week later, a successful performance would be gauged by the same standards. (Roberts postulates that the ability of brain cells (neurons) to adapt to changing conditions is achieved via inhibition of potassium channels. A reduced level of DHEA seems to be a key factor in the debilitating loss of this ability associated with the progression of senile dementia. In support of this contention, he was able to grow brain cells in a tissue culture.)

The rodents with the highest steroid levels performed the best in this maze test. Performance could be enhanced when DHEA was added to the water supply, as well as by direct inoculation. This held true even when the hormone was not received until an hour after the learning experiment had taken place.

J.F. Flood in a 1988 study (*Brain Research*) used mice of various ages and showed that DHEA achieved improvements in memory retention for middle-aged and old mice to the same degree as in young mice.

MEMORY

The classic feature of senile dementia, including Alzheimer's disease, is an inability to remember things, especially at the current time. A patient may very well be able to join in the singing of songs from his youth, fifty years before, but not remember having already sung it and gleefully repeat the same song, time after time for the first time.

DHEA was originally responsible for brain development and can even generate brain cells in the embryonic tissue of a mouse kept in a dish in a laboratory. However, can it revitalize or replace the cells in senile sufferers of these diseases?

One study, by Rudman, involved male nursing-home residents between the ages of fifty-seven and one-hundred-four. Plasma DHEA levels (as one would expect by now?) were inversely related both to clinically identifiable signs of dementia and to the level of assistance required for the activities of daily living. Overall, nursing-home men had low levels of DHEA forty percent of the time. Amongst those requiring total care, this figure rose to eighty percent.

There seems to be little doubt that a lack of DHEA can increase the likelihood of cognitive impairment. The real issue, of course, is whether the addition of DHEA to the diet of older people can restore, or at the very least maintain, brain function to any measurable extent. In fact, some research by Bologa (1987) already substantiates this very point. Supplementation with DHEA prevents neuronal damage.

The Rancho Bernardo Study led by Dr. Barrett-Connor, however, which examined cognitive function was conclusive only for one test and for one gender, women. Barrett-Connor felt that a beneficial effect of DHEA-S, restricted to women and reflective of their better survival, could not be excluded. One could speculate that women are used to lower levels and are able to make more frugal use of the hormone than men. In terms of supplementation, it may merely reflect that men require higher levels of supplementation, in accord with their normative state, than women.

Women also tend to perform better than men, on average, in many cognitive function tests. Cross-gender comparisons, in this instance, are probably not very meaningful.

Concentrations on DHEA in the present study should not be taken to exclude other "smart nutrients" such as gingko biloba for enhancing the activity of blood vessels, or antioxidant vitamins A, C and E in combatting free radicals and consequent oxidation of brain tissue. In combination with hormones such as melatonin and DHEA, they all have an important role to play in maximal brain functioning.

4

The Obesity Connection

FAT LOSS WITHOUT CALORIE REDUCTION

A T THE DANGER OF causing undue excitement, this sub-heading is meant to focus your attention, rather than cause you to rush out and buy DHEA, although this promise is likely to become a common promotion for DHEA. After all, it is a dieter's dream: eat all you want and lose weight. Review the evidence very carefully and decide if you are similar to the profile of the subjects in the study. If so, it may be worth trying.

Obesity is, perhaps, the ideal topic to illustrate the interrelationship of the body and the complex role of DHEA. Current medical terminology classifies obesity as "morbid obesity" because there are so many conditions prevalent in this population besides an excess of adipose tissue. There is usually a whole host of other conditions, several of them with high morbidity rates (i.e., fatal consequences) such as heart disease and diabetes.

Diabetes, heart disease and obesity are interrelated, being risk factors for one another. Besides low levels of DHEA, they each share a common characteristic of elevated blood-sugar levels. DHEA has a beneficial effect on glucose utilization. Of course,

DHEA must be accompanied by other therapeutic measures, notably appropriate caloric intake and activity level.

Animal Studies: Pigs and Dogs

For a change we may review studies involving higher mammals, pigs and dogs.

In his study on boars, conducted for the USDA, Wise (1995) provides a succinct summary of the whole issue of obesity which is applicable to humans. He states that "... so many variables affect obesity (age, genetics, health status) ... new directions, other than reducing or altering diet, are being pursued in controlling obesity in our society."

Wise chose to evaluate the contribution of DHEA using a biological pig model. A major defect in the model is that endogenous DHEA levels derive principally from the testes in pigs and from the adrenal glands in humans (and rats for that matter). Overall, the most meaningful result from the study was the interaction between DHEA and insulin. (This relationship is developed later, in this chapter, as well as under the heading of diabetes.)

Kurzman and MacEwan (1990, 1991) contributed two reports on experiments conducted with dogs. The dogs were fed a range of diets, including high fiber, high fiber and DHEA and DHEA by itself. The high fiber diet produced a substantial reduction in body weight of thirty-one percent. The DHEA diet produced a steady fat loss of four percent per month. The combined high fiber and DHEA diet produced a sixty-six percent fat loss.

Of Mice and Men

A comparable human experiment, by Nestler, with normal weight men treated with DHEA (1,500 mg. daily) produced a similar result (an identical figure), with thirty-one percent fat loss. There was no change in body weight, however, indicating a pound for pound exchange of fatty for lean tissues. Their blood lipids also improved, reducing their risk for heart disease and stroke.

In obese men there is a decrease in both testosterone and DHEA levels as well as an increase of estrogen production. Fat loss with the administration of DHEA helps to restore these hormones to their normal levels. DHEA increases by 125 percent. It may be that endogenous resources can be stimulated and that reliance upon exogenous supplements may be diminished, or even completely discontinued.

With the administration of DHEA there seems to be a reduction in appetite, with a curb on hunger, or a reduced satiety level. It all adds up to eating less without feeling deprived! This may operate via better balance of glucose and insulin levels. One study, in which the rats were given free access to a food supply (*ad libitum,* in the laboratory vernacular) demonstrated a lower food intake. Given the free access, this is interpreted as a voluntary decision. Even so, rats recorded weight loss of fifty percent. In other studies, conducted by another Dr. Yen (Terence T.), rats were able to stay lean without reducing food intake. This is what most people would want: "Have your cake and eat it too"! Dr. Cleary (1984) checked these results on middle-aged rats, bred to have a tendency towards obesity. The rats lost weight when provided with DHEA and the incidence of diabetes also decreased.

Are you confused about these reported changes in food consumption with DHEA usage? Dr. Schwartz was too and undertook some experiments to try and sort it out. He found that the level of dietary fat was the key factor. DHEA-treated rats on a high-fat diet ate less food, while those on a low-fat diet ate more.

People experience similar problems when they attempt to "crash diet." They skip one meal, only to eat more at the next, by which time they are overcome with uncontrollable ravenous urges. They end up eating more at just one meal than they would have consumed in three regular meals spread throughout the day.

Changing from a typical, high-fat American diet to low-fat fruits and vegetables also tends to leave people deprived of essential fatty acids, so that they are doomed to failure within a short time and soon resume their former habits with a vengeance. Such "yo-yo" dieting usually adds on more pounds than they began with, so the general result from improper dieting is fat gain, not fat loss. The word *fat* is used advisedly, since the overall weight may even remain stable, although the exchange from lean to fatty tissues happens in the reverse direction to that mentioned earlier, the reverse of the desired result.

Nevertheless, the work of Schwartz and others has reinforced the promise of DHEA as an anti-obesity agent. Increased appetite, from faulty fat composition, for example, did not negate the benefits of DHEA; and animals still preserved better lean body mass/fat ratios.

Apparently, DHEA inhibits the enzyme (G6PDH — glucose 6-phosphate dehydrogenase) which turns glucose into fat. Dietary sources of fat become important; depending upon which sources are used, alterations in appetite will be reflected. Increased appetite, though, still did not add to the fat stores of the body.

A shift in glucose metabolism from fat production to energy consumption occurs. This may reflect the increased levels of DHEA, or the better sense of well-being, so that high energy leads to higher activity which boosts energy production, and so on. The normal weight males who lost fat while maintaining body weight must have undertaken an increase in activity, although the study did not elaborate upon this aspect. This factor was not controlled because it was unexpected. Just speeding up metabolism would only be expected to burn fat, not build muscle.

Dr. Jonathan Wright (1990) proposes that DHEA produces its anti-obesity effects by inhibiting glucocorticoid activity. Glucocorticoid hormone is also produced by the adrenal glands and stimulates the conversion of surplus glucose to stored glycogen, primarily in the liver. Additionally, DHEA has been shown by Coleman (1984) to play a role in reversing this process, whereby glycogen is available for release from storage and burned for energy by the cells. This reversal is known as "gluconeogenesis."

In obese people, especially those who remain sedentary, circulating levels of blood sugars remain elevated, even when insulin levels increase. There is a delayed sensitivity to insulin production and this eventually fails in many diabetics, who require injections of insulin to maintain normal sugar levels.

DHEA increases sensitivity to insulin, potentiating energy utilization (burning off the glucose). DHEA appears to reduce the need for gluconeogenesis by achieving higher levels of glucose oxidation at the liver. (We will resume this complex discussion of metabolism when we return to the subject of diabetes, later.)

Dr. Schwartz feels that yet another hormone, CCK (cholecytokinin), is the vehicle by which DHEA regulates lean body mass. CCK is the messenger hormone which signals to the brain that the energy intake of food is complete, in other words, "you're full." DHEA seems to facilitate the release of CCK.

Gender Specific Issues

One gender factor may apply, in that the site of storage tends to be gender specific. Women tend to store fat on their hips, men on their abdomen. Furthermore, in women, fat stores surrounding their internal organs (visceral fat) also contribute to circulating sex steroid levels. This was not true for men.

The role of gender was also the focus of attention for Jakubowicz (1995) and his colleagues at the Medical College of Virginia, where the prominent researcher Dr. William Regelson is based. Jakubowicz looked at weight reduction and serum DHEA-S levels in eighteen men and twenty-nine women. Serum DHEA-S was almost double in the women compared to the men. Both groups went on restricted calorie diets. As a result of the weight loss, DHEA-S levels increased by 125% in the men but did not change in the women. Apparently, insulin is responsible for reducing circulating levels of the hormone, but only in men. After two months, when the diet program ended, DHEA-S levels were about the same for both groups.

The Thyroid Connection

We have touched upon adrenal and sex hormones as well as metabolic rates but we have so far left out discussion of another gland, often regarded as the master gland in terms of the body's energy levels: the thyroid. These glands mentioned, together with the pituitary and parathyroid glands, etc., make up the endocrine system, each part of which is sensitive to the other parts.

Many women suffer from cold hands, for example, along with a general inability to feel comfortably warm. This may often be one of the more obvious signs of an undiagnosed hypothyroid condition, i.e., low levels of thyroid hormones. An obese person usually feels hot, being so well insulated. If that person develops diabetes, they tend to develop a new sensitivity to the cold. Previously, they may have been uncomfortably warm at standard room temperatures. Now, they are uncomfortably cold in the same range.

Inadequate thyroid levels may be treated by supplements of iodine and thyroid extracts. Upon initiating DHEA supplements, many women have also found it necessary to make a downward adjustment in their thyroid hormones. Hence, even casually picking up a jar of wild yam cream in order to alleviate PMS symptoms could have repercussions for someone suffering from a thyroid disorder. Hormone manipulation is not a casual affair. It is always wise to discuss supplements, whether natural or not, with pharmacists and physicians. (We will resume our discussion of the thyroid gland elsewhere, including discussion of stress and depression.)

Clearly, a variety of mechanisms is involved, not all of which have been elucidated to date. The bottom line is that DHEA certainly produces fat loss and spares lean body mass.

5

The Sex Connection: Testosterone, Estrogen and Progesterone

THE SELECTION OF TOPICS for chapter headings is a somewhat arbitrary process. The main reason for separate chapters is to reduce the overwhelming amount of information to "bite-size" pieces. It should not be taken to indicate that a particular topic exists in splendid isolation. This applies especially to the current topic: The Sex Connection. If you are following the sequential order of the book, we have already touched upon several aspects of the DHEA hormone as it relates to gender, i.e., male and female variations.

Males have higher levels of DHEA than females: 30:20 mg. respectively, i.e., half as much again; while hormonal fluctuations in the female (both the monthly cycle and the life cycle) tend to be more critically balanced, so that major health problems, like PMS, and problems related to menopause easily fill a chapter of their own. Each of these issues may be seen from the perspective of *gender*, or its synonym: "sex."

Interestingly, an adult male produces more female hormone (estrogen) than a postmenopausal woman; while both men and women become deficient in progesterone after age fifty. So many of our defining standards for the separateness of the sexes become blurred under close inspection. In turn, "sex" also evokes images of coitus and reproduction. If you expected a treatise on human sexuality, however, you will be very disappointed. It is beyond the scope of this book! Suffice to say that there are anecdotal reports of increased libido among male DHEA researchers who have taken the product themselves. One formal study, however, could not confirm this.

More to the point, gender also plays a role in body-fat distribution and body fat, in turn, affects hormonal production. Body fat and hormone levels make a collaborative contribution in the development of certain health conditions, including cancer and diabetes. (These conditions form the basis of other chapters: "The Obesity Connection" and "Immune System Enhancement" and "Therapeutic Uses," respectively. Each of these chapters relates to each of the others, so that there is some duplication of material and overlapping of concepts.)

On one hand, modern medicine is beginning to return to the concept of the patient as a single system, after years of specialization in component parts. On the other hand, whereas most early research on heart disease was conducted solely with male subjects, there is an increasing realization that heart disease among females can exhibit different diagnostic features as well as require unique treatment protocols.

This chapter will deal with the basics of sex hormones but leave detailed consideration of female hormonal dysfunction until the next chapter: "Especially for Women." If a female reader already has a good education in biology she could go directly to that chapter. If the underlying biology becomes too complicated, just refer back to this chapter. This is not a novel, so there is no continuity of plot to worry about.

THE MOTHER HORMONE

While school biology books and the popular media may have imprinted knowledge of certain steroid hormones upon us — usually testosterone for males and estrogen and progesterone for females — DHEA circulates through our bodies in quantities thousands of times greater than either estrogen or testosterone. However, DHEA remained largely forgotten, relegated to the position of a precursor, a "buffer," or reservoir, from which the body could conveniently manufacture more important hormones, as needed, such as: estrogen, testosterone, progesterone and cortisone. Then came the discoveries that not only did many cells in the body actually respond directly to DHEA but that remarkable results were achieved in many experiments using DHEA. A revision of DHEA's importance was called for. Hence, many writers have adopted the term, first coined by Dr. Regelson, that DHEA constitutes the "Mother Hormone."

While DHEA is secreted by the adrenal glands, nearly all of it is converted to DHEA-S (DHEA-Sulfate) which form it takes before circulating throughout the body. The forms are interchangeable and synonymous, for the most part. Supplements are frequently in the form of DHEA-S.

It is worth noting that many reports may not specify the precise form. Some authorities believe that this is remiss, DHEA-S may not be as effective or reliable as DHEA. This is due to the availability of the DHEA. The same holds true for other substances in the body, including minerals and hormones. While there may be adequate levels indicated in a blood test, levels in cells can still be inadequate, owing to an inability to make use of the substance (in this case DHEA).

The transformation of DHEA to DHEA-S (whereby a sulfate is added to the steroid) requires a special enzyme, Dehydroepiandrosterone sulfotransferase (DHEA-ST), which is also produced by the adrenal glands. DHEA-S is the most abundant steroid in circulation in the human and primate and serves as the precursor for the formation of both male and female hormones (androgens and estrogens, respectively). If DHEA is not converted to DHEA-S, the level of DHEA could rise, leading to a mild excess of androgen and associated disorders (e.g., acne).

TESTOSTERONE

Testosterone is well-known as the male hormone, although it is also present in smaller quantities in women. Black women tend to produce higher levels than white women and black men register higher levels than white men, as a group.

Howard (1995) traces the development and survival of the human species to hormonal levels and contrasts the human female with her chimpanzee counterpart. Humans have higher levels of testosterone than chimpanzees, hence their libido is high which enables females to mate outside the limitations of the estrus cycle, in contrast to many lower mammals. The permanent breast display in the human replaces the brief displays of chimpanzees. He cites a study which positively correlated DHEA-S levels with breast development.

DHEA supplementation increases testosterone levels in both men and women.

The concentration of total testosterone (T) declines steeply with age. Zumoff (1995) developed a regression equation [Testosterone (nanomoles per L) = 37.8 x age-1]. Accordingly, the expected testosterone concentration of a woman of forty would be about half that of a woman of twenty-one. Because DHEA and DHEA-S also decline steeply with age, as previously reported, the ratios between DHEA, DHEA-S and T stay the same.

Andropause

Hans Selye is undoubtedly the researcher most responsible for our understanding of the adrenal glands, especially with regard to stress. We have all probably heard of the "fight or flight" response (if we are confronted by a *stimulus* we can stand and fight or turn and run) even if we haven't read Seyle's original works. Also, we are probably well familiar with the concept of stress "burn-out."

Selye viewed the human being from the perspective of his/her inborn survival instincts revealed by chemicals produced instinctively in time of need by the body. For example, if a teacher tells the class they will have a test, the students' heart rates will increase, just as they do before the start of a running race. Or, as they did in ages past when hunting or being hunted. The heart responds to a rush of adrenaline. Nowadays, the stimulus could still be a physical threat such as a close call on the highway, but more typically is simply bad news over the phone. The level of stress is the same, however; both can be fatal, especially when the stress is purely psychological, since the body is stationary and the chemical cocktail is not used up. That is why the highly-stressed businessman can feel better and more relaxed if he schedules some form of exercise. Classically, the stressed businessman will be obese, have high blood pressure, suffer from indigestion and be a candidate for nervous exhaustion, or a heart attack, sooner, rather than later.

If the adrenal glands become *burned out*, they become unable to keep up adequate DHEA production and the health and condition of the individual will suffer, i.e., he or she may seemingly "age overnight." This has been termed the "adrenopause." Given the fact that middle age is also a time of maximum responsibility at work, it may also coincide with the "change of life," termed the *menopause* for women and, sometimes, the *andropause* in men. There is even a relationship between male pattern baldness and DHEA levels. Adrenopause and andropause are similar words; and they may coincide in time, as well as share some similar features.

ESTROGEN

The female gonads (ovaries) are usually stated to produce *estrogen* and progesterone. Both are also produced in men. In fact, estrogen is not an individual hormone but the name of a class of female hormones numbering around twenty, of which three are considered to be major ones: estradiol, estrone and estriol. Each has a particular role to play. Estradiol stimulates breast tissue, with estrone in a supporting role. Estriol is dominant during pregnancy. These hormones determine the higher body fat levels of women. In earlier times this was an advantage for survival.

Now it is generally regarded as a distinct disadvantage. Fat deposition and dietary fats must always be considered within the context of this hormonal link.

The introduction of synthetic estrogens further complicates matters and there is a higher incidence of breast and endometrial cancer (along with other diseases) in population groups of women with a history of oral contraceptive (the Pill) usage. The current trend towards ever-increasing breast cancer rates is frequently linked to the estrogenic effects of industrial pollutants, referred to as "xeno-estrogens."

PROGESTERONE

If estriol is paired with progesterone, as it is during pregnancy, there is a protective effect against breast cancer. During pregnancy, progesterone levels rise to several hundred times their normal peak level, which occurs in the middle of a normal menstrual cycle, prior to ovulation. Inevitably, without ovulation (which includes anovulatory cycles and menopause — surgical, or natural) no progesterone is produced.

Any imbalance in female hormones throws off the entire system, psychologically and physiologically. The very name "hysterectomy" is derived from the removal of *hysteria* (the uterus), the universal medical solution to any *hysterical* female patient.

Physiologically, the "weakest link" may occur anywhere within the endocrine system: pancreas, parathyroid, pituitary, thymus, thyroid, etc., and manifest as diabetes, for example, or gynecological disorders, thyroid disease or psychiatric illness.

An extensive discussion of progesterone is available in a recent book by John R. Lee, M.D.: *Natural Progesterone: The*

Multiple Role of a Remarkable Hormone (Norcross, GA: H.M. Enterprises, 1993). Dr. Lee recommends an over-the-counter natural progesterone skin moisturizer to menopausal osteoporotic patients. He also explains that many other conditions are also largely the result of progesterone deficiency and its attendant estrogen dominance: fibrocystic breast disease, uterine fibroids and PMS.

Menopause

In one study group, the average level of DHEA was 542 in pre-menopausal women, 197 in the postmenopausal group, and 126 in the surgical menopause group whose ovaries had been removed (less than a quarter of normal levels).

Menopause, like andropause, is associated with decreased production and circulating levels of DHEA. In young women DHEA is the resource for about half the female hormones, the other half coming from the ovaries. As the ovaries shut down, there is a dramatic reduction in hormone levels, with consequent symptoms in many women, e.g., hot flashes, which in extreme cases can continue for decades.

With menopause comes increased risk for osteoporosis, which is sometimes the reason physicians prescribe estrogen replacement therapy, although this may increase the patient's chances of breast cancer. Women with higher levels of DHEA-S, in marked contrast to their male counterparts, have been shown in one study, by Barrett-Connor, to suffer an increased risk of death from heart disease.

It is little wonder then that women seek a natural product to ameliorate their symptoms. The Mexican wild yam is widely heralded as the substance women have been waiting for.

(For a complete discussion on Menopause, see the chapter: "Especially for Women".)

At the Shealy Institute (Springfield, MO), blood level indicators of DHEA, like those given for menopause previously, are divided into normal and disease states:

	Ill	Normal	Good	Excellent
Men	180 ng/dl	220 ng/dl	600 - 750 ng/dl	750 - 1250 ng/dl
Women	130 ng/dl	180 ng/dl	450 - 550 ng/dl	550 - 980 ng/dl

A diagnosis may be made just from DHEA levels. Hopefully, restoring DHEA levels through supplementation will also provide some benefit, even if it is not a direct treatment or cure for all diseases.

Osteoporosis

Osteoporosis literally refers to increased porosity in bone, or decreased bone density, as the result of losing calcium; it is understood to effect older women, being related to loss of estrogen. However, elderly men are also involved and should not be ignored.

The emphasis upon studying postmenopausal women has helped to clarify the role of estrogens in bone formation, while the function of androgens in this process remains to be defined. The cells [i.e., human osteoblastic (hOB)] which are responsible for the synthesis and mineralization of bone are now being examined with respect to androgens derived either from the adrenal glands or gonads (of both sexes). Data suggest that DHEA and DHEA-sulfate may play a distinct role in the regulation of human osteoblast function.

DHEA therapy is most widely marketed to appeal to female consumers. They are also the subject of the next chapter: "Especially for Women."

6

Especially for Women: Menopause, Osteoporosis, PMS

MENOPAUSE

M ENOPAUSE IS ASSOCIATED WITH a decline in DHEA Level. Somewhat surprisingly, rather than being purely the result of losing their ovarian component, postmenopausal women with the lowest levels probably have adrenal dysfunction. Other women of the same age may register higher levels of DHEA.

Therapeutically, interest centers around the possibility of achieving a positive response to supplemental DHEA, which was examined in a study by Mortola (1990) at the University of California, San Diego (actually in La Jolla). The data showed that DHEA was rapidly absorbed, and that a prompt conversion to all potent androgens and estrogens occurred, which was sustained for the 28-day duration of treatment. Treatment consisted of four divided doses of 400 mg./day of DHEA. Reassuringly, postmenopausal women retain the ability to transform DHEA. Additionally, DHEA induced insulin resistance and improved lipoprotein (including cholesterol) ratios.

In Mortola's study, DHEA levels did multiply six-fold while estrogens were unchanged, but his population consisted of postmenopausal women.

Certainly, although it is too early to do much more than speculate, the ramifications seem to be promising: that certain menopausal symptoms arising from the deficiency of hormones brought about by ovarian and adrenal cutbacks, may be improved through supplementation. In a premenopausal population, would menopause be delayed? The corollary must also be considered — that restoring hormone levels may also cause unwanted side effects.

OSTEOPOROSIS

Osteoporosis (porous bone) continues as an epidemic, affecting primarily postmenopausal women. Its causes and treatments remain the subject of controversy. Over a million women suffer bone fractures every year. It used to be thought that hip fractures were the result of a fall. It is now thought that the fall is more typically the result of a fracture.

Certainly calcium supplements do not constitute a solution. Many older women lack the ability to absorb calcium even if it is provided. There is a major debate concerning the form of calcium which is the most bioavailable, but this remains academic if there are inadequate gastric juices or vitamin D to make use of it.

Bone formation requires stress (i.e., weight bearing) as well as an appropriate hormonal milieu which is dependent upon the proper functioning of the endocrine system, centering around the parathyroid glands. Since bone mass and serum DHEA both decline with advancing age, sorting out the cause and effect has not been easy. Some studies have been undertaken which are helping to "shed light" upon this issue. Rozenburg (1990) studied a group of Belgian women, finding a significant correlation between bone mineral content and DHEA-S levels, even after correcting for age related changes.

Another study, by Nordin (1985), found that DHEA levels were significantly lower in women with osteoporosis than in a matching age group without osteoporosis.

It is widely agreed that estrogen deficiency is the most significant factor in the acceleration of bone loss which affects many women following menopause. The cells that break down bone (osteoclasts) become more sensitive to the parathyroid hormone. Blood calcium levels rise, which should stimulate the cells that build bone (osteoblasts). However, calcitonin levels are low in postmenopausal women, so excess calcium is excreted. Supplemental calcitonin, derived from salmon, is a promising new therapy. However, it is available by prescription only. One product takes the form of a nasal spray.

Mayer has shown that DHEA affects several of the processes involved in osteoporosis. It stimulates the resorption and formation of bone while inhibiting reabsorption and increasing bone mineral density.

Synthetic estrogen replacement appears to benefit osteoporotic bones in much the same manner, except that its benefits are short-lived (around five years) and there may be a variety of undesirable side effects.

Some authorities make the distinction between early and late phases of the post-menopause, since the ovaries still make a substantial contribution to plasma sex hormones during the initial period. Dr. Vermeulen in Belgium is a leading expert in this field. Essentially, several studies have shown a correlation between adrenal androgens (male hormones produced by the adrenal glands, like DHEA) and bone mineral content. One derivative from DHEA-S (a "metabolite") seems to mimic estrogen, occupying estrogen receptors and inhibiting resorption, but without the constraints of short-lived duration or undesirable side effects.

Mortola studied the effects of DHEA supplementation (1,600 mg. per day). Although estrogen levels were not raised to the levels produced by estrogen therapy (ERT: estrogen replacement therapy), DHEA appeared to be equally effective in preventing osteoporosis. Moreover, DHEA also influenced lipid values in a positive way, which does not occur with estrogen replacement therapy (ERT).

Casson (1995) wanted to demonstrate the bioavailability of DHEA (three weeks of the oral micronized version, 50 mg./d). He got more than he had bargained for: DHEA-S, DHEA, Testosterone, and free Testosterone went to double their premenopausal levels. Upon reflection, he feels that 25 mg./d may be more appropriate.

Another study from Belgium (Rozenberg, 1993) showed that one of the undesirable side effects of estrogen therapy (herein designated as hormone replacement therapy, or HRT), in some cases (20% of their group), is a slight decrease in bone mineral density. This negative effect appeared to occur in women with higher bone mass. Estrogen therapy, then, at best seems to confer a benefit upon women who have a low bone mass at the outset.

Dr. David Williams, another practitioner who champions natural therapies in a newsletter called *Alternatives for the Health*

Conscious Individual, has only positive experiences to report. All postmenopausal women using wild yam cream increased their bone density levels, some by as much as twenty-five percent. Unlike estrogen therapies, this natural compound does more than slow down bone loss. It actually restores bone density and has the added benefit of having no undesirable side effects.

PAIN

It has been noted that Native American women resorted to the wild yam to relieve the pain of childbirth. There has been a recent resurgence of interest in Native American herbal medicine. This has been prompted by several factors, not least the dwindling effectiveness of prescription drugs, which seem to become less effective against pain, in this case, but more likely to produce incapacitating side effects .

Other herbs have become established, particularly in Europe, including "squaw root" (as black cohosh and blue cohosh were commonly referred to). Native Americans also contributed other ideas which are being looked at more closely, as alternatives to C-sections are being explored. The Sioux, for example, utilized an ingenious "squaw belt."

PREMENSTRUAL SYNDROME (PMS)

PMS is often the waste basket term for any physical or emotional symptom suffered by a menstruating woman. Clinically, it should be reserved for a repetitive and predictable condition, directly associated each month with cyclical changes which occur (or fail to occur) in the latter half of the cycle, prior to menses. Supplemental DHEA is believed to relieve this condition through its effect upon circulating LH (luteinizing hormone which stimulates the luteal body — *corpus luteum*) which originates in the pituitary. Women with PMS often have low levels of LH.

Ovulation also triggers the release of progesterone during the second half of the menstrual cycle. Natural progesterone (wild yam cream) boosts progesterone levels, again with positive benefits to the PMS sufferer.

Progesterone appears to be inversely related to estrogen (they have a see-saw relationship, when one goes up, the other goes down and vice versa). Dr. John Lee points out the remarkable similarity between a comprehensive list of PMS symptoms and a compilation of the side effects attendant upon synthetic estrogen therapy. Another list which includes many of the same symptoms can be drawn up for potential side effects associated with synthetic progesterone therapy.

Common symptoms include:
- fluid retention
- headaches
- weight gain
- food cravings
- mood swings

Some symptoms, like fluid retention, may affect individual women differently. Common sites include the breasts and extremities like hands and feet. It is sometimes difficult to differentiate retained fluids from weight gain. Fluid gains can become significant (as much as ten pounds) which encourages many women to avoid drinking and to take diuretics, which disturbs hydration and electrolyte levels, etc., and can be very serious, leading to heart palpitations, panic attacks and high blood pressure much like anorexia.

Leading researchers have also identified nutrient deficiencies, including vitamin B6 (pyrdioxine) and essential fatty acids. GLA derived from the evening primrose is the best known dietary supplement for PMS.

Quite clearly, the same symptoms are produced whenever there is a steroid hormone imbalance. Since DHEA is a precursor of all steroid hormones, any shortage can account for a deficiency, while its renewed availability can restore any deficiencies.

MISCELLANEOUS STUDIES:

Female Athletes

Lindholm (1995) studied the changes in steroid metabolism experienced by female endurance athletes. He concluded that changes in the adrenal production, in favor of glucocorticoid production, is a natural adaptation to sustain blood glucose levels during endurance events.

Other studies have looked at other relationships, including low body fat and menstrual cycle changes, like amenorrhea, which for young athletes can include delayed menarche.

Hirsutism

Exessive body hair in a masculine distribution pattern is thought to be the result of hormonal dysfunction. Measuring total DHEA is a standard means by which androgen overproduction can be traced. Research suggests that DHEA levels, both salivary and blood, are significantly higher in hirsute women. (Vitteck, 1983).

However, this study found a phase-related variation in DHEA levels. Thus, a young woman's DHEA level can only be a valid measurement if it is made relative to the phase of her menstrual cycle (follicular or luteal) and even the rhythms of the day. Phase values were remarkably consistent, although sometimes salivary tests would yield different values than those for plasma. Morning values were triple the afternoon concentrations.

Standardized values are less complicated for postmenopausal women and have been established by Vittek (1983). This confirms that salivary DHEA declines with age.

7

Immune System Enhancement

AIDS, ARTHRITIS, CANCER, CHRONIC FATIGUE SYNDROME, LUPUS

OFTEN WE TEND TO TAKE our good health for granted, little realizing that our immune system is on guard every minute we are alive, and is spurred into a combat mode when faced with disease-causing organisms. As we age, this personal micro-militia becomes less efficient and we become increasingly prone to degenerative disease and aging. As with any other system, the consequences are serious when the immune system malfunctions. It is therefore important to insure that this system is correctly maintained and kept in balance.

Hayfever, rheumatoid arthritis, cancer and other immune-related diseases are on the increase. There is a direct correlation here with our diet, lifestyle and the demands of modern culture, which have all put additional pressure on everyone's immune system. DHEA has been shown to confer special benefits for those suffering from many of these immune-related to "autoimmune diseases." Fortunately, nutritional science has now rediscovered certain natural substances that can be our best form of defense against the onset of many degenerative diseases, as well as from the ravages of pollution and pesticides. These natural substances are called free-radical scavengers, or antioxidants. Along with certain vitamins and minerals, melatonin is among the most potent of antioxidants. To understand free radicals and antioxidants, we need to first look at the immune system.

THE IMMUNE SYSTEM — YOUR PERSONAL FIGHTING FORCE

Contained in the bloodstream, the immune system is made up of many different components, each of which has a highly specific function in protecting the body from attack from outside. The invaders may take the form of chemical pollutants or even heat and cold, and microorganisms such as viruses or bacteria.

The first line of defense against these assailants is the skin, which is our largest organ. The large molecules it contains, as well as the mucous fluids present in the body's openings, have immunological properties and are also acidic. Furthermore, the skin plays host to millions of *friendly* "germs" that fend off *harmful* ones. If an attacking microorganism makes it past the first barrier, it next encounters the phagocytes. These are white blood cells which eat and destroy foreign substances. There are two sorts of phagocyte — the macrophages and the microphages. As their name suggests, macrophages are large cells that surround and eat up dead tissue and cells. If they cannot deal with the enemy, they call for reinforcements. Microphages destroy bacteria.

HOW DOES THE IMMUNE SYSTEM WORK?

Phagocytes provide interim protection until the immune system has marshaled all its forces and is ready to go into operation. Its army comprises specialist organs and cells, and their commander is the thymus gland.

First, there are the leukocytes. These are white blood cells that scavenge the enemy. There are five types of leukocytes — each with a different part to play. The most plentiful of these are the *neutrophils,* which are the first to reach the site of infection.

Eosionophils fight allergies and infections from parasites. They are very active in the later stages of an infection and increase during the healing stages of an inflammation.

Basophils are involved in the battle against blood diseases and some abnormalities of the bone marrow and spinal chord. They are released in chronic inflammation and the healing stages. *Lymphocytes* are the main fighting forces in the leukocyte army. They are formed in the lymph nodes and help to combat viral infections. Last, are the *monocytes,* which fight chronic infection by helping to rid the body of damaged and dead cells. They also prepare body tissue for healing.

Macrophages call on the lymphocytes if they are overwhelmed by the enemy. There are two divisions of lymphocytes — the T-cells and the B-cells. The T-cells are highly specialized cells that fight fungi, viruses and some bacteria, tumors and transplanted cells. There are helper T-cells, suppressor T-cells and cytotoxic T-cells. The helper T-cells secrete a substance called interleukin-2 and this increases the activity of the other T-cells. B-cells are manufactured in the bone marrow and pass through an area in the intestines. They are vital for defending the body against pus-producing bacteria. They break down into plasma cells, which manufacture protein molecules called antibodies, and memory cells. The foreign substances that stimulate the production of antibodies are called antigens.

Antibodies also have another name. They are called immunoglobulins because they are found in the globulin part of blood proteins. There are five types of immunoglobulin. *IgG* is the most important of these. It can squeeze between cells and enter tissue. It neutralizes microorganisms. *IgA* provides immunity for the body's orifices and is present in breast milk (as is *IgG*). *IgM* is the largest of the antibodies and remains in the blood where it kills bacteria, while *IgD* is found almost only in the cell membranes and controls their behavior. *IgE* is responsible for releasing histamines into the blood.

We may sum up the rather complicated immune system in terms of its two principal characteristics. First, it is specific. The immune system is able to recognize an antigen as being foreign. It then reacts by manufacturing specific IgGs. In fact, it can produce millions of different antibodies, each one of which relates to an individual antigen. Once the antibody is produced, the system will make identical antibodies if the same antigen attacks at another time. This is usually what we mean by immunity.

Second, the immune system is also able to recognize when a substance is of the body or when it comes from outside the body, i.e., to distinguish "self" from "non-self." The system stands on guard duty, too, rejecting malignant cells as soon as they appear.

Certain glands and organs are also components of the immune system and they work together with the army of cells. Red bone marrow produces the red blood cells and is the "training ground" for the lymphocytes. It also makes granulocytes, monocytes and platelets for the bloodclotting process. The thymus gland is where the lymphocytes actually originate and it stimulates the development of those cells into plasma cells. Its main function seems to be in the manufacture and export of immunologically competent T-cells to other parts of the body, such as the spleen and the lymph nodes.

The lymphatic system is involved in the collection, filtration and redirection of lymph into the bloodstream and back to the heart. Lymph is the fluid that leaks from the blood through the walls of the tiny blood vessels called capillaries. This fluid bathes the body cells and tissues and provides nourishment in the form of oxygen. The nodes that do the filtering are situated throughout the body. They are the most important source of antibodies and filter bacteria from the lymph stream to prevent the spread of infection.

The spleen is involved in blood formation, storage and filtration. Tonsils act as a filter, protecting against bacteria. The adenoids and the appendix have similar functions.

Free Radicals

It is clear that the body is constantly under attack from microorganisms. Further agents of attack (as if the rest weren't enough for the body to cope with) are free radicals. These are produced when oxygen, or the oxygen component of a substance, is broken down in the process of making energy. However, free radicals need to be kept under control, otherwise they can go on the rampage and start to damage cells and tissues.

Free radicals can come from outside the body. You will remember reading earlier that the immune system protects us not only from microorganisms but also from pollutants. Other similar outside sources may be cigarette smoke, radiation, food additives and certain drugs. If attack from free radicals is prolonged and they are not neutralized, then the immune system may begin to weaken. If the immune system is already weak because the diet has not been supplying the body with the essential nutrients needed to maintain its health — the vitamins, minerals, carbohydrates, proteins and fats in the proper proportions — then illness may result. We may find that we are constantly "coming down" with colds or viruses. Unfortunately, the long-term effects of free-radical damage can include such serious diseases as cancer, heart disease and stroke.

Antioxidants

The way to keep free radicals under control is to consume foods containing antioxidants. Antioxidants are substances that protect the body against free radicals, either by scavenging them or intercepting them within the cell membrane. Well-known antioxidants include vitamins C and E and beta carotene as well as such minerals as selenium and zinc. Research indicates that these antioxidant nutrients help maintain our immune system by protecting against free-radical attack. In view of the fact that deficiency of these nutrients can impair the body's ability to resist disease, experts recommend supplementing the diet with these nutrients.

ENHANCING PROTECTION AGAINST VIRUSES

DHEA has been shown to confer a special protection against viral infections. *The Harvard Health Letter* reported that DHEA added to vaccines helps older mice develop the same vigorous antibodies as young mice.

DHEA has been shown to increase dramatically in response to HIV infection. In 1991, researcher William Regelson reported that people with the HIV virus do not seem to develop full-blown autoimmune disease syndrome (AIDS) until their body's output of DHEA falls. He also found that HIV-positive men with low DHEA levels had double the risk of getting full-blown AIDS compared to those with normal DHEA levels.

Other immune-related diseases which could benefit from DHEA include:
* Rheumatoid arthritis
* Chronic Fatigue Syndrome
* Depression
* Herpes II
* Lupus
* Stress

DHEA has been shown to inhibit virus replication. The antiviral properties of DHEA appear to work via the spleen and thymus gland as well as the adrenals. Bradley set out to determine whether DHEA inhibited replication of feline immunodeficiency virus (FIV) in chronically infected cells. At the concentrations tested, DHEA-S did not inhibit FIV replication or impact on cellular viability or proliferation. [Bradley, W.G.; Kraus, L.A.;

Good, R.A.; Day, N.K. *Vet. Immunol. Immunopathol.* 1995 May; 46(1-2): 159-68.]

Arthritis

The wild yam was used by blacks in the Old South as a potent treatment for rheumatism. Recently, researcher Sambrotk (1988) evaluated DHEA-S in a group of postmenopausal women with rheumatoid arthritis (RA); their levels were significantly lower in comparison with those in healthy controls. While this is exciting, it does not necessarily mean that DHEA-S supplementation would prevent the onset of rheumatoid arthritis, if started early enough, or if DHEA-S is capable of reversing the course of the disease, once it has taken hold. Further research is needed.

One possible explanation for this derives from the traditional use of cortisone-like preparations in the treatment of RA. Cortisone itself was the standard treatment for many years, even with its well-known complications. Many patients were content to suffer the ravages of cortisone, in order to escape the crippling effects of rheumatoid arthritis. However, cortisone weakens the bone matrix and intensifies osteoporosis in women of this age group. Indeed, if they should fracture a hip, the bone may be as soft as an old bathroom sponge, incapable of supporting a prosthetic implant. The individual will need a makeshift joint and be confined to bed, or a wheelchair, with no possibility of ambulation.

Crilly (1979) conducted a study of postmenopausal women under corticosteroid treatment. DHEA (20 mg./day) induced an improved sense of well-being without any adverse side effects.

Even in the absence of cortisone preparations, DHEA levels correlated significantly with bone mineral density. DHEA supplementation in such cases appears worthy of consideration.

Many practitioners report that DHEA can be a valuable adjunct in the treatment of rheumatoid arthritis, and that patients experience less pain, less morning stiffness, increased strength and a reduction in their anti-inflammatory medications.

AIDS

Once again, we are indebted to Howard (1995) for his provocative work in this area, the founding hypothesis of which was formed in 1985. Four years later, supporting evidence for Howard's work came from the orthodox medical community (in the pages of the *Journal of the American Medical Association (JAMA)*, no less). Howard's basic tenet was that since all tissues depend upon DHEA, low levels of DHEA would increase vulnerability to the human immunodeficiency virus. *JAMA* reported that DHEA was found to be low in men infected with HIV and lowest in those progressing to full-blown AIDS.

To reiterate, reduced serum-DHEA levels relate to the development of AIDS. Men with serum-DHEA levels below normal and marginally low T-cell counts (200 - 499) were more than twice (2.34) as likely to progress to AIDS.

In Howard's view, the immune system is underpowered through lack of DHEA. And therefore providing DHEA might offer hope. Oral DHEA was tried (1993) but Howard dismisses these negative results as predictable, since the DHEA would be metabolized as testosterone in the liver, rather than providing freely available levels in the blood. Furthermore, many authorities concur with Howard that there is an inverse relationship between high levels of testosterone and the availability of DHEA.

A refinement in delivery, replacing standard pills, has been achieved through the use of "micronized" (wax-coated) DHEA. This has shown some promise. The desired high blood levels of DHEA have been achieved without increasing testosterone, which might be responsible for some undesirable side effects with standard preparations.

Unfortunately, these formal studies were not conducted with AIDS patients, although in the AIDS underground there has been a great deal of excitement surrounding DHEA, and it is widely available through special channels under provisions accorded these patients by the FDA. Recent work has been undertaken by Henderson (1992), although he found only modest effects.

Further, DHEA is interrelated with another adrenal hormone, cortisol, which enters into the discussion relating to female hormones and diabetes. The immune response operates via the network of lymphatic glands and vessels, under the control of the thymus. Key cells are called lymphocytes. Derived from the thymus gland, they may be designated as T-cells, T-lymphocytes or CD4+, or CD8+, even CD38+.

Lymphocytes respond similarly in a number of potent immune diseases, not just HIV, including: mononucleosis, Epstein-Barr and herpes. Indeed some evidence points to these diseases having a common virus.

T4 (CD4+) counts are a well-known measure of HIV status. Their depletion seems to occur from both the presence of the virus and increased DHEA. Glucocorticoid hormones, on the other hand, in an antagonistic relationship, improve these cell levels, in the short run. Paradoxically, DHEA stimulates the immune system in other ways, including CD8+ and by interfering with glucocorticoid immunosuppression.

All in all it is perhaps a little clearer why the body has such problems with autoimmune diseases. The thymus becomes confused and is unable to distinguish between invading viruses and its own immune cells. People who die from AIDS could be said to be killed by "friendly fire."

The thymus gland shrinks naturally after childhood, although DHEA has been shown to slow this process (Blauer, 1989). A reversal has even been claimed. Since the thymus lies beneath the breastbone, some authorities have recommended the simple procedure of tapping on the breastbone in order to stimulate the gland, through the vibrations. Gerber (1988) has popularized the notion of "vibrational medicine" although this may not be entirely what he had in mind.

Another possible explanation for the efficacy of DHEA is that it also stimulates production of interleukin-2 (which when synthesized, at great expensive, some years back, was considered to be a wonder drug for cancer). This topic will be featured again under the consideration of lupus, although it does appear to have equal application to AIDS.

The most successful pharmaceutical intervention against the development of AIDS has been AZT. Increasingly, AZT has certain disadvantages in some patients and, possibly, against certain strains of the virus. Its benefits seem to depreciate with time and it is proving ineffective against certain strains. Quite likely, as with other synthetic chemicals, some strains may be developing AZT-resistance! DHEA supplementation seems to be helpful, both in reducing replication of AZT-resistant strains, and strains designated as "wild," which never yielded to AZT in the first place.

Breast Cancer

As far back as 1962, researchers in England (Bulbrook, 1962, 1971) reported in *The Lancet* that DHEA was abnormally low in women who developed breast cancer. In a study on 5,000 apparently healthy women, it was found that all twenty-seven of the women who developed and died of breast cancer had blood levels of DHEA less than 10% of the norm for their age group. Furthermore, it took up to nine years before their cancer was diagnosed.

However, DHEA has a dual role in breast cancer. It has been shown to affect the growth of breast cancers too. In humans, very high levels of DHEA and/or dehydroepiandrosterone sulfate (DHEA-S) have been found in breast tissues and secretions which suggest a contributing role in breast cancer growth.

DHEA-S levels in normal breast fluid is many times that found in blood plasma (50 - 1,000 x). This fact has been interpreted in both ways: as a potential inhibitor of breast cancer and a stimulator for it (Regelson).

The body appears to be able to synthesize the hormones best suited to its purpose. Thus, in laboratory animals, DHEA-fed rats had several times more estrogen than controls; they also had less progesterone, which appears to be a co-factor in breast tumor growth. Certainly, in the animal studies, the incidence of mammary tumors and the length of time until the appearance of a tumor, were both improved.

Medical literature from the 1950s to the present establishes the existence of two unrelated abnormalities of androgen production in women with breast cancer. One is the genetically determined presence of subnormal production of adrenal androgens (i.e., DHEA and DHEA-S) in women with premenopausal breast cancer, and their sisters who are at increased risk for breast cancer. The other is excessive production of testosterone, of ovarian origin, in subsets of women with breast cancer (either premenopausal or postmenopausal) and women who are at increased risk for breast cancer, e.g., those with abnormal breast-ducts.

With high testosterone, there is frequently chronic anovulation, which are both characteristic of the polycystic ovary syndrome (PCOS, i.e., multiple cysts on the ovary/ies) that is also frequently seen in women with abdominal ("android") obesity. Both PCOS and abdominal obesity are characterized by a high risk for postmenopausal cancer.

Hormone-sensitive cancers constitute one-third of all cancer cases. These involve the prostate, breast and uterus. Other tissues are classified as steroid producers or "steroidogenic," namely, the ovaries and placenta, testes, adrenals and a large series of peripheral tissues (like body fat). Breast cancer patients with low DHEA levels (both circulating and urinary excretion) generally have a poor outcome (Bulbrook).

Finally, given the use of radiation therapy in breast cancers, DHEA may be useful prophylactically in thwarting undesirable side effects. Wilpart (1986) proposes that DHEA stimulates antimutagenic or DNA repair mechanisms. However, if it is taken too early, it may also make the subject even more sensitive! That is why work is currently being undertaken at the laboratory level.

Chronic Fatigue Syndrome (CFS)

CFS is a catch-all term, classically associated with viral infection, for which there is no definitive protocol which achieves a certain cure. Presumably, stress is a factor, as the disease has been nicknamed "Yuppie flu" in some media. Both CFS and "yuppies" came to prominence in the 1980s.

Recently, a significant number of sufferers have been found to have a chronic form of low blood pressure. Yet again, Howard has a stimulating proposal. In terms of activity levels, he pairs together melatonin and DHEA. Melatonin is widely appreciated as the real "nighttime rest medicine," since blood pressure, heart rate and DHEA are lowered at night. Activity increases blood pressure, heart rate and DHEA levels. Hence, if DHEA levels are marginal, activity could rapidly deplete supplies, so CFS sufferers would have shorter and shorter activity cycles.

This is further compounded by the sleep cycle. CFS sufferers report unrefreshing sleep. They wake up feeling more tired than when they went to bed. Even going back to bed fails to invigorate them. They are *burned out.*

If a viral infection is identified, or suspected, presumably, it achieves its beneficial effects through its anti-viral capabilities. Otherwise, numerous hormonally related imbalances may be restored by the provision of DHEA.

It would appear that a blood test for DHEA levels is required, and if it proves low that the addition of DHEA could effect improvements.

Lupus (Systemic Lupus Erythematosus: SLE)

Lupus is a chronic, inflammatory disease in which the autoimmune system causes numerous abnormalities in blood vessels and connective tissues, including those affecting the skin (rashes), joints (pain), kidneys and nervous system (headaches). Orthodox treatment comprises steroids and chemotherapy, so the "cure" is often worse than the original ill.

A common feature of both murine lupus and human SLE is an interleukin-2 (IL-2) deficiency. While the reason for this remains obscure, recent studies have shown that DHEA raises IL-2 production by the thymus and supplementation dramatically reverses these autoimmune diseases.

Serum samples drawn at the onset of disease, before corticosteroid treatment, also contained low levels of DHEA. Hence, the decreased DHEA levels were not simply a reflection of treatment. Defects of IL-2 synthesis of patients with SLE are at least partly due to the low DHEA activity in the blood.

Preliminary research at Stanford University found that a majority of female patients reported beneficial effects and increased activity levels after receiving DHEA.

DHEA is believed to reduce the production of auto-antibodies, thereby reducing the tendency towards self-destruction.

8

The Stress Connection

MANY PEOPLE RECEIVING DHEA supplements are excited by its effects. They feel younger, they feel better. The ad agency or copy writer might claim that it was a natural, safe version of "Prozac"! We have previously discussed some of the physiological effects of DHEA, mediated via the hormonal system. Peeling back the years automatically makes someone feel better. Yet, there seems to be more to DHEA than that.

DHEA's presence and influence upon the functioning of the brain was discussed in the chapter dealing with the capacity for being "smart." Roberts (1987) postulated that DHEA seems to be a key factor allowing brain cells (neurons) to adapt to changing conditions. He was able to grow brain cells in a tissue culture.

Being younger and more mentally alert takes us to the next level, performing our work more efficiently, feeling up to all of the challenges, which reduces stress, thereby promoting relaxation. It is not surprising, then, why some people are claiming that DHEA is an antidepressant and enhances cognition in those who are majorly depressed .

Literally, as well as figuratively, depression may simply be regarded as a "pit" with no discernible escape route. (Hence: "the pit of depression.") Commonly, another form is widely diagnosed, "manic depression." This consists of oscillations between exuberant optimism and forlorn pessimism. Everything is possible one minute and impossible the next. There is no middle road.

Our society is beset with high stress and, of course, consequently, widespread depression. These two aspects deserve separate consideration, although, like other aspects of the role of DHEA, in reality everything links together. The most eminent authority on "Mind-Body Medicine" is Dr. Deepak Chopra, and he is unequivocal in making the statement that: "DHEA is a marker for the body's exposure to stress."

STRESS

It is convenient to reduce stress to a "fight or flight" response, although life is much more complex these days than in prehistoric times. Physical danger is still a major factor, but day in and day out other sources of stress (i.e., "stressors") tend to dominate. Leading the pack might be emotional worries — beyond the basics of survival — including financial concerns, marital woes and prospects at work. There can be violence in these situations but this is generally the exception rather than the rule.

Ours is also a pervasive drug culture — including the use of tobacco, alcohol, and even caffeine. These are synthetic attempts to boost flagging energy, or "spirits." Unfortunately, many so-called stimulants have a downside, amounting to an "equal and opposite reaction," as in the case of alcohol (in which the old saying: "The morning after the night before..." tells the story).

The scale of one's indulgence tends to change, also. In the beginning, one drink on the way home from work, or one cigarette on the way to work, may achieve the desired effect. That soon becomes two drinks, three drinks, and so on. The source of the stimulus is increased while the effects decrease. At the same time an even more important factor was identified by Dr. Hans Selye (1984). As we adapt to one stressor, we lower our threshold for a new stressor. The cigarette is accompanied by coffee in the morning, the alcohol by a cigarette on the way home in the evening, etc. Additional stressors are required to obtain the desired "adrenaline rush" (specifically norepinephrine). Initially, the additional product produces an effect in very small quantities, or, looked at the other way, the person is likely to receive a disproportionate jolt from average quantities, owing to this sensitization process.

In extreme cases, we may refer to someone's behavior as indicating that she or he is an "adrenaline junkie," always seeking greater thrills. This may come from bigger rides at the fair, or by taking sports, quite literally, to extremes.

In a more moderate sense, physical activity — something as mundane as jogging in the park — can alleviate stress in several ways. Many people find a morning jog, for example, achieves the same benefits as a cup of coffee, without the "downside." They are invigorated for the day.

Other people prefer to "work out" at the end of the day, ridding themselves of the accumulated stresses. They may have been keyed up inside all day at the office, but while their heart may have been pounding, they remained seated in a chair, holding the phone. The "flight" response was in gear, but the body couldn't make use of it. During an evening jog, or competitive game of basketball, the chemical processes can run their full course.

Indeed, after a certain point, the body provides its own chemicals to suppress discomfort — the endorphins. These natural substances lead to "runner's high," or serve to explain why the bruising and stiffness which develops during the basketball game doesn't "hit home" until you reach the showers.

Such natural biochemistry does not have the downside of the synthetic, external substances, as long as it follows its full cycle and supplies of DHEA are adequate to achieve compensation. When DHEA supplies become low, or exhausted, the individual is liable to suffer a nervous breakdown. While physical activity seems to help the hormone balance, it does not do this simply by utilizing DHEA stores. In fact, it seems to boost DHEA levels.

DHEA should not be interpreted as an antidote to stressors, per se. Consuming cups of coffee and smoking cigarettes in place of breakfast to start the day, or a day of yelling on the phone, for example, require other changes and modifications. A nutritious breakfast, less coffee and improved phone etiquette will, however, receive an additional boost from supplementary DHEA.

While our high stress world is also a "high-tech" one, too, this is also more than just coincidence and rhetoric. It is felt that our exposure to the electromagnetic fields emitted by our modern gadgets (computers, phones, radios, televisions, video terminals, etc.) is a level of stress our minds and bodies were not created to withstand. Such exposure is a mild form of radiation and in this respect some benefits have been reported from nutritional supplementation, including DHEA.

DEPRESSION

Dr. Norman Shealy, who operates an institute that bears his name, specializing in mental disorders, reports never having seen a depressed patient with adequate levels of DHEA, nor anyone with adequate levels who is depressed. Quite a clear demarcation!

Therapeutic effects have been reported with dosages of DHEA in the range of 30 - 90 mg. per day. One benefit of this dosage, discernible from blood assays, is an improvement in DHEA levels even among groups of elderly. It seems to be never too late to naturally boost DHEA. (Boosting DHEA is developed further in its own chapter.)

The bottom line is that DHEA is versatile enough to provide the necessary balance for melatonin, which induces restful sleep; and cortisol, which invokes the body's alarm response. Individuals with adequate levels of DHEA can expect the body to handle mental and physical activities at superior levels, without invoking the common signs of burnout, like fatigue, or insomnia ... virtually anything consistent with inferior performance.

9

How To Elevate Your DHEA Levels

BOOSTING ENDOGENOUS LEVELS AND BEST SOURCES (EXOGENOUS): NATURAL OR SYNTHETIC

D HEA IS WIDELY ENDORSED by doctors because it has no alarming toxicity; it is a naturally-occurring substance within the human male and female. And, DHEA supplements are now being recommended by several eminent nutritionists.

Elevating DHEA levels may seem to be the way to go. DHEA is now freely available over the counter, especially at health food stores. The population-at-large has also been delighted to espouse the natural cream, derived from the Mexican wild yam.

In his newsletter *Health & Healing,* Julian Whitaker, M.D. says: "the number of areas in which supplemental DHEA is helpful is almost alarming, because it covers such a broad range of diseases. When blood levels of DHEA are increased to the level you had at a younger age, many diseases just melt away. The body seems fully capable of using supplemental DHEA as if it were processed in the body."

The dosages range usually between 25 and 50 mgs. per day, according to present and hoped-for therapeutic blood levels. A level of 50 mg. per day is normally recommended for the symptoms of aging, although some practitioners are known to use dosages as high as 4000 mg. for specific conditions like multiple sclerosis.

However, it must be understood that DHEA is a powerful hormone which should not be taken indiscriminately. Any dosage in excess of 50 mg. must not be taken without consultation with your health care practitioner.

We can implement certain strategies to boost DHEA levels naturally. In the chapter on stress, the possible contributions of physical exercise and meditation were introduced.

Usually, higher levels of endogenous DHEA have been reported, incidentally, from studies primarily focused on some other aspect of exercise or stress reduction. The studies have not been designed to assess the specific contribution of, e.g., exercise to DHEA production, nor the role of exogenous DHEA in overcoming some existing deficiency, caused by an adrenoandrogen condition.

The Shealy Institute innovated one particular therapeutic modality designed, specifically, to enhance DHEA production in the presence of a variety of conditions, e.g., diabetic neuropathy, PMS and rheumatoid arthritis. This modality consists of a form of electro-acupuncture, whereby acupuncture points determined to be associated with the condition are stimulated, without the use of needles. Dr. Shealy reports a reduction of pain syndromes and, of greater significance for our present topic, DHEA production increased by as much as fifty-six percent.

Interventions need not be as innovative, nor as technical as this. One tack is to avoid those factors which reduce the DHEA reservoir. Alcohol and tobacco should spring immediately to mind. Women, especially, need to carefully monitor their intake of synthetic hormones, for contraception or hormone replacement, for example. These depress normal hormone production and functioning.

Speaking of mind, it is important to stay calm, avoiding the negative impact of stress upon DHEA levels. A well-balanced lifestyle is the best way to summarize this and several other components of the DHEA-conservation approach. This includes maintaining ideal weight and lean body mass, which demands moderate eating, as well as a good night's rest.

On a more pro-active note, some of these same factors do more than just conserve DHEA levels, they can have a positive contribution as well. Practicing relaxation, such as meditation, has boosted recorded levels. Glaser (1992) has been the principal researcher in this area. He looked at DHEA levels in a large group of experienced meditators, specifically practitioners of Transcendental Meditation (TM). DHEA levels, above the norms for the same age and gender in control groups of non-meditators, correlated almost perfectly in the female population, with significant (eight of eleven groups) correlation for men.

Given the linear fall in levels of DHEA normally associated with age, these higher levels were also interpreted by Glaser as evidence of an age reversal, so to speak. In Glaser's estimation, the gains were in the order of five or ten years.

While age might be anticipated to win out eventually, when studying the effect of meditation on DHEA levels the results went in the opposite direction — the biggest differences showed up in the older subjects. An attempt was made to control for several notable factors, like diet, exercise, alcohol consumption and body weight. It is somewhat speculative to make any profound statements about the skill of meditation (which would be expected to increase with experience and age) relative to the degree of stress each group of subjects is subjected to (which might be anticipated to decline in terms of a comfortable lifestyle, for example, but increase with stressful events like deaths of parents and other loved ones, or declining faculties).

Glaser's "older" group were only forty-five years old. The meditating men enjoyed DHEA levels twenty-three percent higher than controls. The women were even more impressive, fully forty-seven percent more. Sonka (1968) has noted that the age in which DHEA deficiency is identifiable is between forty and fifty. From this perspective, Glaser's group was well chosen.

BEST SOURCES

There is only one natural source of DHEA — the Mexican wild yam (Dioscorea). This form may also be designated as "diosgenin." Doubt has been expressed concerning the efficacy of yam products in elevating serum levels. The most popular form is as a topical cream. Concentrations of progesterone in the cream are stated to be 450 mg. per ounce. Positive results are frequently reported, mostly anecdotally. Contemporary and traditional uses have been primarily by women for the range of female problems. Yet, boosting progesterone levels in men has also been associated with health benefits for certain conditions.

Another form called Colloidal DHEA is administered sublingually and composed of particles that are ultrafine: 0.0001 to 0.01 microns in diameter. This is supposed to assure the best absorption and use by the body. These ultrafine particles do not dissolve but remain suspended in a suitable electrically-charged liquid (demineralized water). DHEA is present in ionized form which makes it biologically available at an instant!

SAFETY, INTERACTIONS AND CONTRAINDICATIONS

Thankfully, in marked contrast with some listings in the Physician's Desk Reference (PDR) for pharmaceuticals, DHEA warrants a scant section.

Safety

The Shealy Institute in Springfield, MO is a major center with respect to the prescription of DHEA. Dr. Shealy has not commented upon, nor is he aware of any existing literature detailing any significant complications of DHEA supplementation. A mild form of acne and slight hirsutism are the only conditions worth mentioning.

Dr. Shealy has stated, categorically, that there are no reported side effects from diosgenin, extracted from the Mexican wild yam.

Contraindications

Conditions which may be found to represent contraindications, even though this is still a precaution, rather than a reaction, comprise hormonally-based cancers, i.e., breast, ovary or uterus cancer in women, and prostate cancer in men.

10

Therapeutic Uses / Research Briefs

BURNS

PROGRESSIVE ISCHEMIA AND NECROSIS of the skin following thermal injury are reduced by post burn administration (subcutaneous injection) of DHEA of the steroid hormone DHEA.

DHEA reduces progressive dermal ischemia caused by thermal injury. Araneo, B.A.; Ryu, S.Y.; Barton, S.; Daynes, R.A. *J. Surg. Res.* 1995 Aug; 59(2): 250-62.

CANCERS

All cells must replicate themselves in order to maintain life. However, some cells can go on multiplying, completely out of control, eventually consuming the rest of the body. This condition is known as cancer and may occur in any area of the body. The underlying mechanisms of both normal and abnormal replication are poorly understood. Certainly, however, the most prominent candidates include:

- exposure to the sun, or other forms of radiation (including x-rays);
- toxins, like cigarette smoke and pesticides; and even
- viruses and parasites (e.g., pancreatic fluke — Clark, 1993).

Tobacco is regarded as responsible for almost one-third of all cancers, by far the largest single contribution of any factor. The next largest source is believed to be natural aflatoxins found in foods, including peanuts.

Age is one factor which may simply be the cumulative effect of one form of exposure or another. Gender is inextricably linked to some cancers, which are gender specific, e.g., ovarian and prostate. Breast cancer probably comes to mind, but the breast is not a primary sexual factor; it is a secondary one. Hence, just as some men may develop rudimentary breasts, some men may also develop breast cancer. The proportions are, of course, infinitesimally small; women sustain some ninety-nine percent of breast cancers.

DHEA has shown great promise during animal studies. DHEA has inhibited tumor development, prevented breast cancer from developing and provided some impunity against carcinogens in food. Research has firmly established that low levels of DHEA exist in association with a number of cancers:

- Bladder (Gordon)
- Breast (Bulbrook, 1971)

- Gastric (Gordon)
- Prostate (Stahl, 1992)

One key to DHEA's success in suppressing overactive cellular proliferation is the enzyme G6PDH, which we've mentioned elsewhere when discussing cholesterol and diabetes. High G6PDH activity is observed in precancerous and cancerous cells. Blockage of these activities, by DHEA, would inhibit carcinogen synthesis (Van Noorden, 1984), including the growth of a tumor (Feo and Pascale, 1990).

Depending upon the stage at which the cancer is exposed to additional levels of DHEA, the direct contributions of DHEA supplementation include:

- slows oxidation;
- reduces free radical formation;
- slows proliferation of precancerous tissue;
- interrupts tumor development;
- speeds repair of, e.g., radiation damaged cells.

Other factors are also influential, dependent upon the age, gender and health of the subject (diabetic, for example). These include:

- inhibition of fat formation;
- boosts androgen formation;
- suppresses overproduction of other hormones, i.e., restores hormonal homeostasis.

The hormonally-responsive tumors affecting the breast are considered separately, under the section: "Especially for Women."

However, breast cancer does deserve to be included in any purportedly all-inclusive list of cancers which have been shown to respond to DHEA administration so far in laboratory studies. The type of cancer and the relevant author are provided in the accompanying list:

- Breast (Viral: Schwartz, 1993)
- Breast (Radiation-induced: Inano, 1995)
- Colon (Schultz, 1991)
- Lung (Pashko, 1981)
- Lymphatic (Risdon, 1990)
- Skin (Pashko, 1981)

Of course, it is not intended to imply that taking DHEA will effect a cure or provide immunity from these cancers. The best protection from lung cancer is not to smoke, yourself, or inhale anyone else's "second-hand smoke." The most sensible way to avoid skin cancer is to dress appropriately and stay out of the sun.

The use of DHEA, especially in the form of a topical cream, to stimulate hormones in cases of this type of cancer is questionable. If the cancer is hormonally related, hormonal stimulation may be contraindicated. Others may feel that the restoration of hormone balance through the addition of DHEA is precisely what is required.

We will probably have to rely upon the usual serendipity of scientific advance, whereby a group of women, using the cream, may have undiagnosed and unsuspected cancers, which will be in a state of remission when a diagnostic screening is undergone; or aggravate the condition. In the current litigation climate in the U.S., no sponsor is forthcoming for this type of research.

CRYPTOSPORIDIOSIS

Cryptosporidiosis is a diarrheal disease in humans and other animals caused by the coccidian parasite, Cryptosporidium parvum.

Boosting the immune system by exogenous DHEA may be useful in the treatment of cryptosporidiosis.

DIABETES

Diabetes encompasses a host of complex metabolic processes which are interdependent and interrelated. Several fields of research concentrate upon these processes. Essentially, diabetes is a state whereby the body cannot regulate the balance between glucose and insulin, related to energy. We may formally refer to a maladapted response. This may also be viewed as a reaction to stress: "fight or flight." Stress can play a role in diabetes but it is the physiological, rather than the psychological, aspects which are of primary concern for the moment.

Many authorities believe that the initial maladaptation is a state of hypoglycemia, which may be even more clearly defined using the original term: hyperinsulinemia. There is an overproduction of insulin, causing low blood sugar. This destroys the pancreas (or, in some views, the pancreas is being destroyed by an infection, either viral or parasitic) which creates a hypoinsulinemic state, such that glucose is elevated with no endogenous system to control it. Hence the reliance upon insulin injections.

Nestler (1994) gives credence to the simple view that, since aging and obesity are both characterized by insulin resistance and a decline in DHEA, DHEA may be the principal factor at work. However, as Buffington points out, adrenocortical activity may underlie the development of diabetes in women, as the genders react differently.

In both pre- and postmenopausal women, androgenic (i.e., male) hormones are associated with insulin resistance and hyperinsulinemia. According to Buffington (1994), adrenocortical activity may underlie the development of diabetes in women. They have the opposite effect in men — increased testosterone and DHEA levels lower insulin concentrations.

When all is said and done, assuming sex change is not a therapeutic option, even after adjustment for age, obesity and body fat distribution, Haffner (1994) found (for men) that insulin retained an inverse correlation with free testosterone, total testosterone and DHEA. Thus, low testosterone and low DHEA levels indicated low insulin levels. Moreover, free testosterone and DHEA exhibit inverse correlations with glucose concentrations. Thus, when glucose is high, testosterone and DHEA are lower and vice versa, when testosterone and DHEA are high, glucose is lower.

The major role accorded to DHEA in some quarters derives from its ability to inhibit glucose 6 phosphate dehydrogenase. This is expanded upon under the cholesterol subheading in the section on heart disease.

The world of mice has generously contributed a special strain which loses pancreatic cells during its lifetime. Upon receiving DHEA, these beta cells were preserved and the trend towards developing diabetes in these mice was reversed. In a related experiment, (Coleman, 1984) mice with diabetes were given DHEA and the severity of the disease was reduced.

FIBROBLASTS

DHEA and its sulfate derivative (DHEA-S) reportedly have anti-diabetic and anti-obesity effects. To elucidate the underlying mechanism/s, the effect of DHEA was examined on glucose uptake in cultured human fibroblasts. Results suggested that DHEA increases Glut-1 mRNA through binding to a specific factor in cultured human fibroblasts and thereby stimulates glucose uptake in these cells (Nakashima, 1995).

INSULIN GROWTH FACTOR (IGF-I)

IGF-I is considered to be one of the most important growth factors during puberty. Information concerning its correlation to thyroid hormones (T3, T4), adrenal and sex steroids is limited to puberty and the elderly. Hesse (1994) assembled a group of subjects, who ranged in age from newborn to one-hundred years. Increasing adrenal DHEA-S concentrations stimulates IGF-I synthesis and by means of gonadal steroidogenesis, increases the pubertal GH secretion and the further pubertal IGF-I increase. The low IGF-I concentrations in patients over sixty years reflect the more catabolic metabolism of the elderly.

INSULIN RESPONSE

Nestler (1991) set out to determine whether a reduction in insulinemia would be associated with a rise in serum dehydroepiandrosterone (DHEA) sulfate in insulin-resistant men. He was able to conclude that benfluorex treatment lowers blood pressure, improves glucose tolerance, reduces the glucose-stimulated insulin response and increases serum DHEA and DHEA sulfate in both middle-aged and elderly men.

The significance of an insulin imbalance (insulin resistance and insulin levels) hold true in non-diabetic patients. The presence of hyperinsulinemia and insulin resistance is also a constant occurrence with all major cardiovascular risk factors. Heart disease, in turn, further impairs glucose handling. We will explore this relationship further, under the heading of heart disease. Unfortunately, for the morbidly obese diabetic with heart disease, the bottom line is premature death. Only the precise details need to be filled in. Ultimately, saving the heart at the expense of the kidneys will be fatal. As will saving the kidneys at the expense of the heart. Checkmate!

HEART DISEASE

In spite of some signs of improvement, heart diseases remain the number one cause of death in the United States and most other Western nations. Though men appear to be more prone, any protective factor for women is undermined by the presence of diabetes and hypertension.

Hypertension, you may recall, reflects arterial blockage and correlates with cholesterol and DHEA levels. This continues to hold true if the conditions deteriorate to the point of a myocardial infarction (heart attack). LaCroix has confirmed that patients for whom the attack was fatal had lower levels of DHEA than those who survived. Slowinska's retrospective study (1989) found that low levels existed months after the attack.

The association between DHEA and coronary disease did not hold true for women, in the study by Herrington (1995).

According to a study published in the *New England Journal of Medicine* (1986), Elizabeth Barrett-Connor, M.D. (University of California School of Medicine in San Diego) observed DHEA levels in 242 men (ages 50 to 79) for twelve years. In men with a history of heart disease DHEA levels were significantly lower than in men with no history of heart disease. Further, Barrett-Connor and other researchers concluded that even in people without heart disease, DHEA seems to protect against early death.

Treatment

Now let's turn to the question of whether supplements with DHEA are an antidote, helping to buffer patients from premature heart failure, or actually reversing the progression of atherosclerosis and associated conditions (hypertension, angina etc.)?

At John Hopkins Medical Institute, rabbits with severe arteriosclerosis were treated with DHEA, resulting in an almost 50% reduction in plaque size.

Individuals with higher DHEA sulfate have a much lower risk of heart disease.

It has been postulated that DHEA and its sulfate ester (DHEA-S), the major secretory products of the adrenal gland, may be discriminators of life expectancy and aging.

DHEA-S levels decreased with age and were also significantly lower in men with a history of heart disease than in those without such a history. The decrease was 6 - 7 micrograms per deciliter (similar to the 5 - 6 by Orentreich, 1980). The 50th percentile may be placed at 140 micrograms per deciliter.

Data (from Haffner, 1995) suggest that the DHEA-S concentration is independently and inversely related to death from any cause, and death from cardiovascular disease in men over age fifty.

CHOLESTEROL

High concentrations of lipoprotein Lp(a) have been related to atherosclerotic disease, both at coronary and cerebrovascular levels. Although Lp(a) levels are under a strict genetic control, being inversely related to the molecular weight of apo(a) isoforms, an interference of endogenous sex steroids on Lp(a) metabolism has been hypothesized, positively and independently related to LDL-cholesterol and DHEA-S

Data (Denti, 1994) suggest that endogenous testosterone and estradiol do not affect Lp(a) metabolism in males, at least in physiological concentrations. However Lp(a) might be affected by DHEA-S, the most abundant product of the adrenal gland.

Estrogen use has been reported to decrease triglyceride and low-density lipoprotein cholesterol (LDL-C) and increase high-density lipoprotein cholesterol (HDL-C). In both pre- and postmenopausal women, several studies have shown that increased glucose and insulin concentrations are associated with increased free testosterone and decreased sex hormone-binding globulin.

In contrast, increased androgen concentrations in men do not seem to be associated with increased cardiovascular risk factors, although testosterone concentrations are associated with increased HDL-C and decreased insulin concentrations. DHEA and dehydroepiandrosterone sulfate (DHEA-S) appear to be associated with improved cardiovascular risk factors in men, but this connection in women is less clear.

Studies with respect to the lowering of cholesterol levels have been more explicit. Supplements with oral DHEA-S have reduced total serum cholesterol levels by an average of eighteen percent (Haffa, 1994). We may recall from the section on body fat that this decrease does not require a change in diet or activity level. Several mechanisms have been proposed. Suffice to say that DHEA and cholesterol are intimately connected, including in the literal sense, as LDL (low density lipoprotein) is the major DHEA transporter in blood. However, this does not mean to imply that the two are positively correlated. In fact, the relation is more positive (in the sense of encouraging) in that they are inversely correlated. When DHEA levels rise, cholesterol levels fall.

While cholesterol is essential in the body, it is regarded with paranoia because of its association in the negative processes of arterio- and atherosclerosis. As long as cholesterol levels are balanced, it is not a problem. It is thought that the cholesterol itself undergoes some transformation, to render it more "sticky" both to itself and the arterial walls. In addition, damage to the arterial walls seems to facilitate the initial deposition. Several amino acids are implicated together with the enzyme G6PDH (glucose 6 phosphate dehydrogenase). This produces the oxidation and release of free radicals we hear so much about these days.

By blocking this enzyme, DHEA also reduces the creation of free radicals and spares the arterial walls. Remember, when there is sufficient DHEA to go around, it rides along with the cholesterol, so it is readily available to exert control over these processes. In its absence, things go awry.

FATTY ACID METABOLISM

It is well established that DHEA treatment is associated with an increase in fatty acid metabolism. This condition would require levels of L-carnitine much higher than those physiologically present in the liver. The possibility thus exists that during DHEA treatment the concentration of L-carnitine may become a limiting factor for fatty acid oxidation and therefore responsible for some of the effects observed after administration of the hormone.

BIBLIOGRAPHY

Abbasi, A., Mattson, D.E., et al., Hyposmatomedinemia and hypogonadism in hemiplegic men who live in nursing homes. *Arch. Phys. Med. Rehabil.* 1994 May; 75(5): 594-599.

Adinoff, B., Martin, P.R., Eckardt, M.J., Linnoila, M., Role of DHEA and DHEA-S in Alzheimer's disease. *Am. J. Psychiatry* 1993 Sep; 150(9): 1432-3.

Aizawa, H., et al., Androgen status in adolescent women with acne vulgaris. *J. Dermat.* 1995, 22(7): 530-532.

Anapliotou, M.G., Sygrios, K., et al., Adrenal hyperresponsiveness to ACTH stimulation in women with polycystic ovary syndrome; an adrenarchal type of response. *J. Clin. Endocrinol. Metab.* 71(4), 1990 Oct; 900-906.

Aradhana, R., Kale, R.K., Diosgenin-a growth stimulator of mammary gland of ovariectomized mouse. *Indian J. Exp. Biol.* 30(5), 1992 May; 367-370.

Araneo, B.A., Ryu, S.Y., Barton, S., Daynes, R.A., Dehydroepiandrosterone reduces progressive dermal ischemia caused by thermal injury. *J. Surg. Res.* 1995 Aug; 59(2): 250-62.

Argtielles, A.E., et al., Endocrine profiles and breast cancer. *Lancet*, 1973; 1: 165-168.

Barrett-Connor, E., Rhaw, K.T., Yen, S.S.C., A prospective study of dehydroepiandrosterone sulfate, mortality, and cardiovascular disease. *N. Eng. J. Med.* 1986; 315:1519-1524.

Barrett-Connor, E., Edelstein, S.L., A prospective study of dehydroepiandrosterone sulfate and cognitive function in an older population: 'The Rancho Bernardo Study.' *J. Am. Geriatr. Soc.* 42(4), 1994 Apr.; 420-423.

Barrett-Connor, E., et al., A prospective study of dehydro-epiandrosterone sulfate (DHEAS) and bone mineral density in older men and women. *Am. J. Epidemiol.* 1993, 137(2): 201-206.

Battelli, D., et al., Effects of dehydroepiandrosterone and carnitine treatment on rat liver. *Biochem. Mol. Biol. Int.* 1994, 33(6): 1063-1071.

Baulieu, E.E., Studies on dehydroepiandrosterone (DHEA) and its sulphate during aging. *C. R. Acad. Sciences II* 1995, 318(1): 7-11.

Beaton, G., Practical population health indicators of health and nutrition. *WHO Monograph*, 62(1976); 500.

Becker, U., Gluud, C., et al., Menopausal age and sex hormones in postmenopausal women with alcoholic and non-alcoholic liver disease. *J. Hepatol.* 1991 Jul; 13(l):25-32.

Belanger, B., Belanger, A., Labrie, F., *J. Stero. Biochem.* (32), 1989; 695-698.

Belanger, B., Caron, S., Belanger, A., Dupont, A., Steroid fatty acid esters in adrenals and plasma: effects of ACTH. *Clin. Chem.* 36(12), 1990 Dec; 2042-2046.

Belanger, A., et al., Changes in serum concentrations of conjugated and unconjugated steroids in 40- to 80-year-old men. *J. Clin. Endocrin. Metab.* 1994, 79(4): 1086-1090.

Bell, H., Raknerud, N., et al., Inappropriately low levels of gonadotrophins in amenorrhoeic women with alcoholic and non-alcoholic cirrhosis. *Eur. J. Endocrinol.* 1995 Apr; 132(4): 444-9

Berkenhager-Gillesse, E.G., et al., Dehydroepiandrosterone sulphate (DHEA-S) in the oldest old, aged 85 and over. *Ann. N. Y. Acad. Sci.* (719), May 31, 1994; 543-552.

Bernstein, L., Relationship of hormones use to cancer risk. Exogenous hormones are widely prescribed in the United States, primarily as oral contraceptives and hormone replacement therapy. *Monog. Natl. Cancer. Inst.* 1992-1 (12): 137-147.

Blauer, K.L., et al., *Proc. Am. Soc. Endocrinol.*, Abs. (25), 1989; 29.

Bologa L., Sharma, J., Roberts E., DHEA and its sulfate derivative reduce neuronal death and enhance astrocytic differentiation in brain cell cultures, *J. Neurosci. Res.* 1987; 17:225-234.

Bolt, H.M., Interactions between clinically used drugs and oral contraceptives. *Environ. Health Perspect.* 1994 Nov; 102 Suppl 9: 35-8

Bradley, W.G., Dehydroepiandrosterone inhibits replication of feline immunodeficiency virus in chronically infected cells. *Vet. Immunol. Immunopathol.* 1995, 46(1-2): 159-168.

Braverman, E. R., DHEA and Adrenopausea; A New Sign of Aging and a New Treatment, *Total Health*, 1995, 16:1.

Brignardello, E., et al., Dehydroepiandrosterone concentration in breast cancer tissue is related to its plasma gradient across the mammary gland. *Breast Cancer Res. Treat.* 1995, 33(2): 171-177.

Browne, E.S., et al., Dehydroepiandrosterone: Antiglucoconicoid action in mice. *Am. J. Med. Sci.* 1992; 303: 366-371.

Buffington, C.K., Givens, J.R., Kitbachi, A.E., Enhanced adrenocortical activity as a contributing factor to diabetes in hyperandrogenic women. *J. Endocrinol.* 140(2), 1994 Feb; 297-307.

Bulbrook, R.D., Hayward, J.L., Spicer, C.C.F., Relations between urinary androgen and corticoid excretion and subsequent breast cancer. *Lancet* (2) , 1971: 395-8.

Calabrese, B.P., Isaacs, E.R., Regelson, W., Dehydro-epiandrosterone in multiple sclerosis: positive effects on fatigue syndrome in a non-randomizing study. In: *The Biological Role Of Dehydroepiandrosterone.* (Edited by M. Kalimi and W. Regelson), New York: de Gruyter, 1990; 95-100.

Carlstrom, K., Stege, R., Adrenocortical function in prostatic cancer patients: effects of orchidectomy or different modes of estrogen treatment on basal steroid levels and on the response to exogenous adrenocorticotropic hormone. *Urol. Int.* 45(3), 1990; 160-163.

Carmina, E., Lobo, R.A., Pituitary-adrenal responses to ovine corticotropin-releasing factor in polycystic ovary syndrome and other hyperandrogenic patients. *Gynecol. Endocrinol.* 4(4), 1990 Dec; 225-232.

Carmina, E., et al., Reassessment of adrenal androgen secretion in women with polycystic ovary syndrome. *Obstet. Gyn.* 1995, 85(6): 971-976.

Casson, P.R., et al., Replacement of dehydroepiandrosterone enhances T-lymphocyte insulin binding in postmenopausal women. *Fertil. Steril.* 1995, 63(5): 1027-1031.

Castagnetti, L., Short report on the 5th symposium on the analysis of steroids. *Steroids* 59(l), 1994 Jan; 55-56.

Cayen, M.N., Dvomick, D., Effect of diosgenin on lipid metabolism in rats. *J. Lipid Res.* 20(2), 1979 Feb; 162-167.

Chopra, D. *Perfect Health: The Complete Mind Body Guide.* New York: Crown Publishing, 1991.

Cistemino, M., Transdermal estradiol substitution therapy for the induction of puberty in female hypogonadism. *J. Endocrinol. Invest.* 1991 Jun; 14 (6): 481-488.

Clark, Hulda R., *Cure for All Cancers*, San Diego: ProMotion Publ., 1993.

Cleary, M.P., Shepherd, P., Jenits, B., Effect of dehydroepiandrosterone on growth in lean and obese Zucker rats. *J. Nutr.* 1984; 114:1242-1251.

Clerici, M., Bevilacqua, M., Vago, T., et al., An immunoendocrinological hypothesis of HIV infection. *Lancet* 343(8912), June 18, 1994; 1552-1553.

Coleman, D.L., Laiter, E.H., Applerweig, N., Therapeutic effects of dehydroepiandrosterone metabolities in diabetes mutant mice. *Endocrinology*, 1984; 115, 239-243.

Colgan, M., Fielde, S., Colgan, L.A., Micronutrient status of endurance athletes affects hematology and performance. *J. Appl. Nutr.* Vol (43), No. 1, 1991; 17-36.

Comstock, G.W., et al., The relationship of serum dehydroepiandrosterone and its sulfate to subsequent cancer of the prostate. *Cancer Epidemiol. Biomarkers. Prev.* 1993, 2(3): 219-221.

Conget, J., et al., Evaluation of clinical and hormonal effects in hirsute women treated with keto conazole. *J. Endocrinol. Invest.* 13(11), 1990 Dec; 867-870.

Crilly, R.G., Marshall, D.H., Nordin, B.E.C., Metabolic effects of corticosteroid therapy in postmenopausal women. *J. Steroid Biochem.* 1979; 11:429-433.

Culig, Z., Hobisch, A., et al., Mutant androgen receptor detected in an advanced-stage prostatic carcinoma as activated by adrenal androgens and progesterone. *J. Immunol.* 152(7), 1994 Apr 1; 3417-3426.

Cummings, D.C., Androgenesity and androdynamics in normal women. *Cleve. Clin. J. Med.* 57(2), 1990 Mar-Apr; 161-166.

Dean, W., *Smart Drugs and Nutrients*. Petaluma, CA: Health Freedom, 1991.

De la Torre, B., et al., Relationship between blood and joint tissue DHEAS levels in rheumatoid arthritis and osteoarthritis. *Clin. Exp. Rheumatol.* 1993, 11(6): 597-601.

de Lignieres, B., Transdermal dihydrotestosterone treatment of "andropause." *Ann. Med.* 1993 Jun; 25(3): 235-241.

Denti, L., et al., Correlations between plasma lipoprotein Lp(a) and sex hormone concentrations: a cross-sectional study in healthy males. *Horm. Metab. Res.* 1994, 26(12): 602-608.

Derogatis, L.R., Rose, L.I., Shulman, L.H., et al., Serum androgens and psychopathology in hirsute women. *J. Psychosm. Obstet. Gynaecol.* 14(4), 1993 Dec.

Dettling, M., Heinz, A., et al., Dopaminergic responsivity in alcoholism: trait, state, or residual marker? *Am. J. Psychiatry* 1995 Sep; 152(9): 1317-21

Deuster, R.A., et al., Nutritional intakes and status of highly trained and amenorrheic women runners. *Fertil. Steril.* (46), 1986; 636.

Devogelaer, J.P., Crabbe, J., DeDeuxchaisnes, C.N., Bone mineral density in Addison's disease: Evidence for an effect of adrenal adrogens on bone mass. *Br. Med. J.* 1987; 294: 798-800.

Diamonti-Kandarakis, E., et al., Raptis-S insulin sensitivity and antiandrogenic therapy in women with polycystic ovary syndrome. *Metabolism* 1995, 44(4): 525-531.

DiBlasio, A.M., et al., Maintenance of cell proliferation and steroidogenesis in cultured human fetal adrenal cells chronically exposed to adrenocorticotropic hormone: rationalization of in vitro and in vivo findings. *Biol. Reprod.* 42(4), 1990 Apr; 683-691.

Doldin, B., Estrogen excretion patterns and plasma levels in vegetarian and omnivorous women. *N. Engl. J. Med.* 307, 1982; 1: 1542.

Drocker, W.D., Blumberg, J.M., et al., Biologic activity of dehydroepiandrosterone sulfate in man. *Journal of Clinical Endocrinology,* 1972; 35, 48-50.

Ebeling, P., Koivisto, V.A., Physiological importance of dehydroepiandrosterone. *Eng. J. Clin. Endocrinol. Metab.* 78(6), 1994 Jun; 15-20.

Ehrmann, D.A., Rosenfield, R.L., Hirsutism beyond the steroidogenic block. *N. Engl. J. Med.* 323(13), 1990 Sept 27; 909-911.

Eisen, A., Et al., Dehydroepiandrosterone sulphate (DHEAS) concentrations and amyotrophic lateral sclerosis. *Muscle Nerve,* 1995, 18(12): 1481-1483.

Enzi, G., et al., (eds.), *Obesity: Pathogenesis and Treatment.* New York: Academic Press, 1981.

Erenus, M., et al., Comparison of the efficacy of spironolactone versus flutamide in the treatment of hirsutism. *Gynecol. Endocrinol.* 7(4), 1994 Dec.

Faasati, P., Fassati, M., et al., Treatment of stabilized liver cirrhosis by dehydroepiandrosterone. *Agressologia* 14(4), 1973; 259-268.

Falany, C.N., et al., Human dehydroepiandrosterone sulfotransfrerase. Purification, molecular cloning and characterization. *Ann. N. Y. Ac. Sciences* 1995, 774: 59-72.

Feo, F., Pascale, R. Glucose-6-phosphate dehydrogenase and the relation of DHEA to carcinogenesis. In: *Biological Role of DHEA.* NewYork: de Gruyter, 1990, 397-404.

Flood, J.F., et al., *Brain Research* 1988 (488), 178-181.

Gaby, A., *Preventing and Reversing Osteoporosis*. Rockwell, CA: Prima Publishing, 1994; 157-172.

Gavaler, J.S., Alcohol effects on hormone levels in normal post-menopausal women and in postmenopausal women with alcohol- induced cirrhosis. *Recent Dev. Alcohol* 1995;12: 199-208

Gavaler, J.S., et al., Hormonal status of postmenopausal women with alcohol-induced cirrhosis: further findings and a review of the literature. *Hepatology* 1992 Aug; 16(2): 312-319.

Gerber, Richard. *Vibrational Medicine: New Choices for Healing Ourselves*. Santa Fe: N.M.: Bear and Co. Publishing, 1988.

Gilad, S., Chayen, R., Tordjman, K., et al., Assessment of 5 alpha-reductase activity in hirsute women: comparison of serum androstanediol glucuronide with urinary androsterone and aeticholanolone excretion. *Clin. Endocrinol.* (Oxf) 1994, 40(4): 459-464.

Gladstar, R., *Herbal Healing for Women*. New York: Simon and Schuster, 1993; 183-258.

Glaser, J.L., et al., Elevated serum DHEA sulfate levels in practitioners of TM and TM siddhi program. *Journal of Behav. Medicine* 1992, 15(4):327-34.

Gordon, G., et al., Reduction of atherosclerosis by administration of dehydroepiandrosterone. *J. Clin Invest.*, Department of Medicine, Johns Hopkins Medical Institutions, 1988 Aug; 82(2): 712-720.

Haffa, A.L., et al., Hypocholesterolemic effect of exogenous dehydroepiandrosterone administration in the rhesus monkey. *In Vivo* 1994 Nov-Dec; 8(6): 993-997.

Haffner, S.M., et al., Decreased testosterone and dehydroepiandrosterone sulfate concentrations are associated with increased insulin and glucose concentrations in nondiabetic men. *Metabolism* 1994, 43(5): 599-603.

Haffner, S.M., Valdez, R.A., Endogenous sex hormones: impact on lipids, lipoproteins and insulin. *Am. J. Med.* 1995, 98 (1A): 40S-47S.

Hakkinen, K., Pakarinen, A., Serum hormones and strength development during strength training in middle-aged and elderly males and females. *Acta. Physiol. Scand.* (Finland) 1994 Feb; 150(2): 211-219.

Harvard Health Letter. DHEA gets respect. July, 1994.

Henderson, E., Yang, J.Y., Schwartz, A., Dehydroepiandrosterone (DHEA) and synthetic DHEA analogs are modest inhibitors of HIV- I IIIB replication. *AIDS Res. Hum. Retroviruses* 1992 May; 8 (5): 625-31

Herrington, D.M., Dehydroepiandrosterone and coronary thrombosis. *Ann. N. Y. Ac. Sciences* 1995, 774: 271-280.

Hesse, V., et al., Insulin-like growth factor I correlations to changes of the hormonal status in puberty and age. *Exp. Clin. Endocrinol.* 1994; 102(4): 289-98.

Hill, M., Gut bacteria and aetiology for cancer of the breast. *Lancet* 2, 1971; 472.

Hill, P., Plasma hormones and lipids in men at different risk for coronary heart disease. *Am. J. Clin. Nutr.* 22, 1980.

Howard , M. J., DHEA, Melatonin and Testosterone in Human Evolution. *DHEA Home Page,* http//www.napleas.net. 1995

Inano, H., Ishii-Ohba, H., Suzuki, K., et al., Chemoprevention by dietary dehydroepiandrosterone against promo-progression phase of radiation-induced mammary tumorigenesis in rats. *J. Steroid Biochem. Mol. Biol.* 1995 Jul; 54(1-2): 47-53.

Ito, D., *Without Estrogen: Natural Remedies for Menopause and Beyond.* New York: Carol Southern Books, 1994.

Iwasaki, M., Darden, T.A., Parker, C.E., Tomer, K.B., Pedersen, L.G., Negishi, M., Inherent versatility of P450 oxygenase. Conferring dehydroepiandrosterone hydroxylase activity to P450 2a-4 by a single amino acid mutation at position 117. *Breast Cancer Res. Treat.* (3), 1990 Oct, 16; 261-272.

Jacobson, M.A., et al. Decreased derum dehydroepiandrosterone is associated with an increased progression of human immunodeficiency virus infection in men with CD4 cell counts of 200-499. *J. Infect. Disease.* 1991: 164: 864-868.

Jakubowicz, D.J., et al., Disparate effects of weight reduction by diet on serum dehydroepiandrosterone-sulfate levels in obese men and women. *J. Clin. Endocrinol. Metab.* 1995, 80(11): 3373-3376.

Jesse, R.L., et al., Dehydroepiandrosterone inhibits human platelet aggregation in vitro and in vivo. *Ann. N. Y. Ac. Sci.* 1995, 774: 281-290.

Josephs, J.A., Roth, G.S., Whitaker, J.R., In: *Intervention In The Aging Process. Part 2,* (W. Regelson and N. Sinex, eds.) New York: Alan R. Liss, 1983; 187-202.

Juarez-Oropeza, M.A., Diaz-Zagoya, J.C., Rabinowitz, J.L., In vivo and in vitro studies of hypocholesterolentic effects of diosgenin in rats. *Int. J. Biochem.* 19(8), 1987; 679-683.

Kalimi, M., Regelson, W., (eds.), *The Biologic Role of Dehydroepiandrosterone (DHEA).* New York: W. de Gruyter, 1990.

Khalil, M.W., Strutt, B., Vachon, D., et al., Effects of dexamethasone and cytochrome P450 inhibitors on the formation of 7 alpha-hydroxydehydroepiandrosterone by human adipose stromal cells. *J. Steroid Biochem. Mol. Biol.* 48 (5-6), 1994 Apr; 545-552.

Khoury, M.Y., Barachat, E.C., Pardini, D.P., Vieira, J.G., Delima, G.R., Serum levels of androstanediol glucuronide, total testosterone, and free testosterone in hirsute women. *Atherosclerosis* 105(2), 1994 Feb; 191-200.

Kirchner, M., The role of hormones in the etiology of human breast cancer. *Cancer* 39, 1977; 2716.

Koo, E., Fehr, K.G., Fehr, T., Fust, G., *Klin. Woehenschr.* (61), 1983; 715-717.

Krieg, M., Nass, R., Tunn, S., Effects of aging on endogenous level of 5 alphadihydrotestosterone, testosterone, estradiol, and estrone in epithelium and stroma of normal and hyperplastic human prostate. *J. Clin. Endocrinol. Metab.* 1993 Aug; 77(2): 375-38.

Kundu, A.K., Sharma, A.K., A rapid screening technique for detection of diosgenin through in situ cytophotometry. *Stain Technol.* 63(6), 1988 Nov; 369-372.

Kurzman, I.D, et al., Reduction in the body weight and cholesterol in spontaneously obese dogs by DHEA. *Int. J. Obesity*, 1990, 14:95-104.

Labrie, F., et al., *[Intracrinology. Autonomy and freedom of peripheral tissues].* (In French.) *Ann. Endocrinol.* Paris, 1995, 56(1): 23-29.

Lardy, H., Stratinan, F., *Hormones, Thermogenesis and Obesity.* New York: Elsevier, 1988, 337-452.

Lee, John R.M., M.D., *Natural Progesterone: The Multiple Role of a Remarkable Hormone.* Norcross, GA: H.M. Enterprises, 1993.

Lewis, D.A., Anti-inflammatory drugs from plant and marine sources. *Agents Actions Suppl.* (27), 1989; 373.

Lindholm, C., et al., Altered adrenal steroid metabolism underlying hypercortisolism in female endurance athletes. *Fertil. Steril.* 1995, 63(6): 1190-1194.

London, B.M., Lookingbill, D.P., Frequency of pregnancy in acne patients taking oral antibiotics and oral contraceptives. (letter) *Arch. Dermatol.* 1994 Mar; 130(3): 392-3.

Loviselli, A., et al., Low levels of dehydroepiandrosterone sulfate in adult males with insulin-dependent diabetes mellitus. *Minerva Endocrinol.* 1994 19(3): 113-119.

Luu-The,V., et al., Structural characterization and expression of the human dehydroepiandrosterone sulfotransferase gene. *DNA Cell. Biol.* 1995,14(6): 511-518.

MacEwan, G.E., Kurzman, I.D. Obesity in the dog: role of the adrenal steroid DHEA. *J.Nutr.* 1991, 121:51-55.

Majewska, M.D., Demirgoren, S., Spivak, C.E., London, E.D., The neurosteroid dehydroepiandrosterone sulfate is an allostericantagonist of the GABAA receptor. *Brain Res.* 526(i), 1990 Aug 27; 143-146.

Malinow, M.R., et al., Effects of synthetic glycosides on steroid balance in Macac afascicularis. *J. Lipid Res.* 28(l), 1987 Jan; 1-9.

Marrero, M., Prough, R.A., Frenkel, R.A., Milewich, L., Dehydroepiandrosterone feeding and protein phosphorylation, phosphatases, and lipogenic enzymes in mouse liver. *Exp. Clin. Endocrinol.* 96(2), 1990 Nov; 149-156.

Matsumoto, A.M., "Andropause" — are reduced androgen levels in aging men physiologically important? *West. J. Med.* 1993 Nov; 159(5): 618-620. Comment on: *West. J. Med.* 1993 Nov; 159 (5): 579-585.

Mayer, D., Weber, E., Bannasch, P., Modulation of liver carcinogenesis by dehydroepiandrosterone. In: *The Biological Role of Dehydroepiandrosterone* (Kalimi, M. and Regelson, W., eds.) New York: de Gruyter, 1990; 361-385.

Merril, C.R., Hanrington, M.G., Sunderland, T., Reduced plasma dehydroepiandrosterone concentrations in HW infections and Alzheimer's disease. In: *The Biological Role of Dehydroepiandrosterone* (Edited by Kalimi, M., and Regelson, W.) New York: de Gruyter, 1990; 101-105.

Meyer, J.H., Gruol, D.L., Dehydroepiandrosterone sulfate alters synaptic potentials in areas of CAI of the hippocampal slice. *Maturitas* 17(3), 1993 Nov; 205-210.

Midgley, P.C., Azzopardi, D.N., Shat, J.C., Honour, J.W., Virilisation of female preterm infants. *Arch. Dis. Child* 65 (7 Spec No.), 1990 Jul; 701-703.

Miklos, S., Dehydroepiandrosterone sulphate in the diagnosis of osteoporosis. *Acta. Biomed. Ateneo. Parmense.* 1995, 66 (3-4): 139-146.

Monroe, S.E., Menon, K.M.J., Changes in reproductive hormone secretion during the climacteric and postmenopausal periods. *Clin. Obstet. Gynecol.* 1977; 20:113-122.

Moore, N., *The Facts About DHEA: Bountiful Health, Boundless Energy, Brilliant Youth.* Dallas, Texas: Charis Publishing Co., Inc., 1994.

Morales, A.J., et al., Effects of replacement dose of dehydroepiandrosterone in men and women of advancing age. *J. Clin. Endocrinol. Metab.* 1994, 78(6): 1360-1367.

Moran, C., et al., Heterogeneity of late-onset adrenal 3 beta-ol-hydroxysteroid dehydrogenase deficiency in patients with hirsutism and polycystic ovaries. *Arch. Med. Res.* 1994, 25(3): 315-320.

Mortola, J.F., and Yen, S.S.C., The effects of oral dehydroepiandrosterone on endocrine-metabolic parameters in postmenopausal women. *J. Clin. Endocrinol. Metab.* 1990; 71: 696-704.

Murphy, S., Khaw, K.T., Cassidy, A., Compston, J.E., Sex hormones and bone mineral density in elderly men. *Bone Miner.* 1993 Feb; 20(2): 133-140.

Nakashima, N., et al., Effect of dehydroepiandrosterone on glucose uptake in cultured human fibroblasts. *Metabolism* 1995, 44(4): 543-548.

Nawata, H., Tanaka, S., Tanaka, S., et al., Aromatase in bone cell: association with osteoporosis in postmenopausal women. *J. Steroid. Biochem. Mol. Biol.* 1995 Jun; 53(16): 165-174.

Nestler, J.E., Strauss, J.R., Insulin as an effector of human ovarian and adrenal steroid metabolism. *Endocrinol. Metab. Clin. North Am.* 1991 Dec; 20(4): 807-823.

Nestler, J.E., Clore, J.N., Blackard, W.G., Metabolism and actions of dehydroepiandrosterone in humans. *J. Steroid Biochem. Mol. Biol.* 1991; 40(6): 599-605.

Nestler, J.E., Clore, J.N., Blackard, W.G., Dehydroepiandrosterone: the missing link between hyperinsulinemia and atherosclerosis? *FASEB J.*, 1992 Sept; 6(12): 3073-3075.

Nestler, J.E., McClanahan, M.A., Diabetes and adrenal disease. *Baillieres Clin. Endocrinol. Metab.* 1992 Oct; 6(4): 829-847.

Nestler, J.E., Beer, N.A., Jukubowicz, D.J., Beer, R.M., Effects of a reduction in circulating insulin by metfonmin on serum dehydroepiandrosterone sulfate in nondiabetic men. *J. Clin. Endocrinol. Metab.* 1994 Mar; 78(3): 549-554.

Nestler, J.E., et al., Effects of insulin reduction with benfluorex on serum dehydroepiandrosterone (DHEA), DHEA sulfate and blood pressure in hypertensive middle-aged and elderly men. *J. Clini. Endocrinol. Metab.* 1995, 80(2): 700-706.

Nishi, Y., Nonclassical 3 beta-hydroxysteroid dehydrogenase deficiency in young girls with hirsutism and premature pubarche. *Endocrinol. Jpn.* 37(5), 1990 Oct; 763-767.

Nordin, B.E.C., et al., The relation between calcium absorption, serum dehydroepiandrosterone, and vertebral mineral density in postmenopausal women. *J. Clin. Endocrinol. Metab.* 1985; 60: 651-657.

Odumosu, A., Wilson, C.W., Hypocholesterolemic effects of vitamin C, clofibrate and diosgenin in male guinea-pigs [proceedings]. *Br. J. Pharmacol.* 67(3), 1979 Nov; 456P-457P.

Orentreich, N.J., et al., Age changes and sex differences in serum dehydroisoandrosterone (DHA) and dehydroisoandrosterone sulfate (DHAS) and the DHA to DHAS ratio in normal adults. *J. Clin. Endocrinol. Metab.* 1980, 51: 330-333.

Orlandi, F., et al., Estrone-3-sulfate in human breast cyst fluid. Relationship to cition-related cyst subpopulations. *Ann. N. Y. Acad. Sci.* 586, 1990; 79-82.

Oskai, L.B., The role of exercise in weight control. In: *Exercise and Sport Science Reviews*, Vol 1, (Wilmore, J.H., ed.) New York: Academic Press, 1975, 105-123.

Paczkowski, C., Wojciechowski, Z.A., The in vitro synthesis of diosgenin mono- and diglucoside by enzyme preparations from Solanum melongea leaves. *Acta. Biochim. Pol.* 40(l), 1993; 141-143.

Parker, L., *Adrenal Androgens in Clinical Medicine.* New York: Academic Press, 1988.

Parough, R.A., Webb, S.J., Wu, H.Q., Lapenson, D.P., Waxman, D.J., Induction of microsomal and peroxisomal enzymes by dehydroepiandrosterone and its reduced metabolite in rats. *Cancer Res.* 54(11), 1994 Jun 1; 2878-2886.

Pashko, L.L., Schwartz, A.G., Agou-Gharbia, M., Inhibition of DNA synthesis in mouse epidermis and breast epithelium by DHEA related steroids. *Carcinogenesis* (2), 1981, 717-721.

Perrone, L., et al., Endocrine studies in children with myelomeningocele. *J. Pediatric. Endocrinol.* 1994, 7(3): 219-223.

Purohit, A., Howarth, N.M., Potter, B.V., Reed, M.J., Inhibition of steroid sulphatase activity by steroidal methylthiophosphonates: potential therapeutic agents in breast cancer. *Metabolism* 43(5), 1994 May; 599-603.

Reed, M.J., Purohit, A., Duncan, L.J., et al., The role of cytokines and sulphatase inhibitors in regulating oestrogen synthesis in breast tumours. *J. Steroid. Biochem. Mol. Biol.* 1995 Jun; 53(1-6): 413-20.

Reff, M.E., Schneider, E.L., *Biological Markers in Aging.* Bethesda, MD: NIH Pub., 1980; 82.

Regelson, W., Loria, R., Kalimi, M., Hormonal intervention: buffer hormones or state dependency. The role of dehydroepiandrosterone (DHEA), thyroid hormone, estrogen and hypophysectomy in aging. *Ann. N. Y. Acad. Sci.* 1988; 521: 260-273.

Regelson, W., Loria, R., Kalimi, M., Dehydroepiandrosterone (DHEA) the mother steroid. Immunologic action. *Ann. N. Y. Acad. Sci.* (719), May 31, 1994; 553-563.

Remer, T., Fintelmann, A., Manz, F., Measurement of urinary androgen sulfates without previous hydrolysis: a tool to investigate adrenarche. Determination of total 17 ketosteroid sulfates. Report of the National Institute of Health Expert Panel on Weight-loss. Meeting in Bethesda, MD, 31 March-2 April 1992.

Risdon, G., Cope, J., Bennett, M., Mechanisms of chemoprevention by dietary dehydroisoandrosterone. Inhibition of lymphopoiesis. *Am. J. Pathol.* 1990 Apr; 136(4): 759-69.

Rittmaster, R.S., Thompson, D.L., Effects of leuprolide and dexamethasone on hair growth and hormone levels in hirsute women: the relative importance of the ovary and the adrenal in the pathogenesis of hirsutism. *J. Clin. Endocrinol. Metab.* 70(4), 1990 Apr; 1096-1102.

Roberts, E., Effects of dhea and its sulfate on brain tissue in culture and memory of mice. *Brain Res.* 1987, 406: 357-362.

Rosen, T., Hansson, T., Granhed, H., Szucs, J., Bengtsson, B.A., Reduced bone mineral content in adult patients with growth hormone deficiency. *Acta. Endocrinol.* (Copenhagen), 1993 Sept; 129(3): 201-206.

Rosen, T., Eden, S., Larson, G., Wilhelmsen, L., Bengtsson, B.A., Cardiovascular risk factors in adult patients with growth hormone deficiency. *Acta. Endocrinol.* (Copenhagen), 1993 Sept; 129(3): 195-200.

Rowland, D.L., Greenleaf, W.J., Dorfman, L.J., Davidson, J.M., Aging and sexual function in men. *Arch. Sex. Behav.* 1993 Dec 22; (6): 545-557.

Rozenberg, S., et al. Age, steroids and bone mineral content. *Maturatis* 1990; 12: 137-143.

Sadowsky, M., Antonovsky, H., Sobel, R., Maoz, B., Sexual activity and sex hormone levels in aging men. *Int. Psychogeriatrics* 1993 Fall; 5(2): 181-186.

Sambrotk, R.N., et al., Sex hormones status and osteoporosis in postmenopausal women with rheumatoid arthritis. *Arthritis Rheum.* 1988; 31: 973-978.

Sasagawa, I., Satomi, S., Effects of high-dose medroxyprogesterone acetate on plasma hormone levels and pain relief in patients with advanced prostatic cancer. *Br. J. Urol.* 65(3), 1990 Mar; 278-281.

Schmidt, J.B., Lindmaier, A., Spona, J., Endocrine parameters in acne vulgarism. *Endocrinol. Exp.* 24(4), 1990 Dec; 457-464.

Schubert, W., Cullberg, G., Edgar, B., Hedner, T. Inhibition of 17 beta-estradiol metabolism by grapefruit juice in ovariectomized women. *Maturitas* 1994 Dec; 20(2-3): 155-163.

Schulz, S., Nyce, J.W., Inhibition of protein isoprenylation and p2 I ras membrane association by dehydroepiandrosterone in human colonic adenocarcinoma cells in vitro. *Cancer Res.* 1991 Dec 15; 51(24): 6563-7

Schwartz, A.G., Pashko, L.L., Cancer chemoprevention with the adrenocortical steroid dehydroepiandrosterone and structural analogs. *J. Cell. Biochem. Suppl.* (17G), 1993; 73-79.

Schwartz, A.G., Fairman, D.K., et al., The biological significance of dehydroepiandrosterone. *Carcinogenesis* (10), 1988; 1809.

Schwartz, A.G., Inhibitions of spontaneous breast cancer formation in female C3H(Avy'a) mice by long-term treatment with dehydroepiandrosterone. *Cancer Res.* 1979; 39: 1129-1132.

Schwartz, A.G., Pashko, L.L., Mechanism of cancer preventive action of DHEA. Role of glucose-6-phosphate dehyrdogenase. *Ann. N. Y. Ac. Sci.* 1995, 774: 180-186.

Selye, Hans, M.D., *The Stress of Life.* New York: McGraw Hill, 1984.

Slowinska, S. J., et al., Decreased Plasma DHEA Sulfate and Dihydrostestesterone Concentrations in Young Men after Myocardial Infarction. *Atherosclerosis* 1989, 79:197-203.

Sonka, J., et al., Serum lipids and dehydroepiandrosterone excretion in normal subjects. *J. Lipid Res.* 9, 1968; 769-772.

Stahl, F., Schnorr, D., Pilz, C., Dorner, G. DHEA Levels in Patients with Prostatic Cancer, Heart Disease and Under Surgery Stress. *Exp. Clin. Endocrinol.* 1992; 99(2): 68-70.

DHEA: The Ultimate Rejuvenating Hormone

Sun, X. R., Risbrider, G.P., Site of macrophage inhibition of luteinizing hormone stimulated testosterone production by purified leydig cells. *Biol. Reprod.* 50(2), 1994 Feb; 363-367.

Sunderland, T., et al., DHEA and Alzheimer's disease. *Lancet (2),* 1989; 570.

Suzuki, T., et al., Low serum levels of dehydroepiandrosterone may cause deficient IL-2 production by lymphocytes in patients with systemic lupus erythematosus (SLE). *Clin. Exp. Immunol.* 1995, 99(2): 252-255.

Taelman, P., et al., Persistence of increased bone resorption and possible role of dehydroepiandrosterone as a bone metabolism determinant in osteoporotic women in late postmenopause. *Maturitas,* 1989; 11:65-73.

Thewles, A., Parslow, R.A., Coleman, R., Effect of diosgenin on biliary cholesterol transport in the rat. *Biochem. J.* 291 (Pt3), 1993 May 1; 793-798.

Terzolo, M., et al., Adrenal incidentaloma, a five year experience. *Minerva Endocrinol.* 1995, 20(1): 69-78.

Uchida, K., Takase, H., Nomura, Y., Takeda, K., et al., Changes in biliary and fecal bile acids in mice after treatments with diosgenin and beta-sitosterol. *J. Lipid Res.* 25(3), 1984 Mar; 236-245.

Valimaki, M., Pelkonen, R., et al., Pituitary-gonadal hormones and adrenal androgens in non-cirrhotic female alcoholics after cessation of alcohol intake. *Eur. J. Clin. Invest.* 1990 Apr; 20(2): 177-81.

Van Noorden, C.J., Vogels, I.C.M., Houtkooper, J.M., et al., Glucose -6, phosphate dehydrogenase activity in individual rat hepatocytes of different ploidy classes. *Eur. J. Cell Biol.* (33), 1984; 157-162.

Vilette, J.M., et al., Circadian variations in plasma levels of hypophyseal, adrenocortical and testicular hormones in men infected with human immunodeficiency virus. Comment in: *J. Clin. Endocrinol. Metab.* 70(3), 1990 Mar; 563-565, 572-577.

Wade, C.E., Lindberg, J.S., Cockerell, J.L., et al., Upon admission adrenal steroidogenesis is adapted to the degree of illness in intensive care unit patients. *J. Clin. Endocrinol. Metab.* 67, (2) 1988; 223-227.

Whitaker, J., *Health and Healing Newsletter.* Potomac, MD: Phillips Publishing Inc. To order: (301-424-3700).

Williams, D. *Alternatives for the Health Conscious Individual.* Ingram, TX: Mountain Home Publ., (PO Box 829, Ingram, TX 78025.) To order: (1-800-527-4044).

Wilpart, M., Speder, A., Ninane, P., Roberfroic, M., Antimutagenic effects of natural and synthetic hormonal steroids. *Teratogenesis, Carcinogenesis, Mutagenesis.* (6), 1986; 265-273.

Wise, T., Klindt, J., Buonomo, F.C., Obesity and dehydroepiandrosterone/dehydroepiandrosterone sulfate relationships in lean, obese, and meat-type cross-bred boars: responses to porcine growth hormone. *Endocrinology* 1995 Aug; 136(8):3310-7.

Wright, Jonathan, *Dr. Wright's Guide to Healing with Nutrition.* New Canaan, CT: Keats Publ., 1990.

Yang, J.Y., Schwartz, A., Henderson, E.E., Inhibition of 3'azido-3'deoxythymidine-resistant HIV- I infection by dehydroepiandrosterone in vitro. *Biochem. Biophys. Res. Commun.* 1994 Jun 30; 201(3): 1424-32

Yang, J.Y., Schwartz, A., Henderson, E.E., Inhibition of HIV-1 latency reactivation by dehydroepiandrosterone (DHEA) and an analog of DHEA. *AIDS Res. Hum. Retroviruses* 1993 Aug; 9(8): 747-54

Yen, S.S., et al., Effects of replacement dose of dehydroepiandrosterone in men and women of advancing age. *J. Clin. Endocrinol. Metab.* 1994 Jun; 78(6): 1360-7.

Yen, T.T, et al., Prevention of obesity in Avy'a mice by dehydroepiandrosterone. *Lipid* 1977; 12: 409-413.

Zumoff, B., et al., Abnormal 24-hr mean plasma concentrations of dehydroepiandrosterone and dehydroepiandrosterone sulfate in women with inoperable breast cancer. *Cancer Res.* (41), 1981; 3360-3363.

Zumoff, B., et al., 24-hour mean plasma testosterone concentration declines with age in normal premenopausal women. *J. Clin. Endocrinol. Metab.* 1995, 80(4): 1429-1430.

AUTHOR PROFILE

Hasnain Walji, Ph.D. is an expert consultant on natural health and a researcher and writer specializing in nutrition and complementary therapies. He is the author of *Live longer/ Live Healthier: The Power of Pycnogenol* (Hohm Press, 1996), *The Vitamin Guide-Essential Nutrients for Healthy Living*, published by Element Books, and six books as part of a new series exploring common ailments from complementary and orthodox points of view published by Hodder Headline Plc. and endorsed by the Natural Medicine Society of England. The titles are: *Asthma and Hayfever, Skin Problems, Addiction, Headaches & Migraine, Arthritis & Rheumatism and Heart Health*. The series has been translated into Spanish.

Dr. Walji's other tiles include *Vitamins, Minerals and Dietary Supplements: A definitive Guide to Healthy Eating* published by Hodder Headline. *Using Aromatherapy at Home*, published by C.P.R. Publishing, Cleveland, UK. He has also written a series of books for Thorsons-Harper Collins for their "Nutrients for Health" series. The titles include, *Melatonin; Vitamin C; Bee Products;* and *Folic Acid.*

A contributor to several journals on environmental and Third World consumer issues, Hasnain Walji was the founder and editor of "The Vitamin Connection - an International Journal of Nutrition, Health and Fitness," published in the UK, Canada and Australia, focusing on the link between health and diet. He also launched "Healthy Eating," a consumer magazine focusing on the concept of optimum nutrition, and has written a script for a six-part television series, "The World of Vitamins," to be produced by a Danish Television company.

Dr. Hasnain Walji is the Program Director of Software Development Innovations, Inc. (Dallas, Texas), the publishers and developers of "The Natural Health Information System"™ which comprises of an interactive suite of programs called NutriPlus™ and Health Plus.™ He lives and works in Dallas, Texas.

INDEX

parathyroid gland   41, 47
phagocyte   54, 55
pineal gland   2
pituitary gland   15, 16, 41
PMS (Pre-Menstrual Syndrome)   34, 42, 49–51
polycystic ovary syndrome   65
postmenopausal   42, 43, 45, 46, 47, 49, 52
premenopausal   42, 46, 48
preventative medicine   17
progesterone   2, 36, 37, 40, 41, 42, 50, 64
Prozac   68
psychiatric illness   41

R
rashes   66
REM   24
rheumatoid arthritis   15, 53, 59, 60, 61

S
schizophrenia   23, 24
self repair   15
senile dementia   22, 25, 26
sexual dysfunction   20
SIDS (Sudden Infant Death Syndrome)   23

sleep   16
sleep disorders   2
sports nutrition   9
stress   13, 39, 40, 59, 68–71
stroke   30, 58

T
testosterone   1, 2, 37, 38, 39, 48, 65
thymus   41, 63
thyroid   34, 41, 55
toxins   12
trauma   16

U
uterine fibroids   42

V
varicose ulcers   15
vibrational medicine   63

W
weight gain   50
weight loss methods   9
wild yam cream   49, 50

ADDITIONAL TITLES OF INTEREST FROM HOHM PRESS

10 ESSENTIAL HERBS, REVISED EDITION
by Lalitha Thomas

Peppermint. . .Garlic. . .Ginger. . .Cayenne. . .Clove. . . and 5 other everyday herbs win the author's vote as the "Top 10" most versatile and effective herbal applications for hundreds of health and beauty needs. *Ten Essential Herbs* offers fascinating stories and easy, step-by-step direction for both beginners and seasoned herbalists. Learn how to use cayenne for headaches, how to make a facial scrub with ginger, how to calm motion sickness and other stomach distress with peppermint, how to make slippery-elm cough drops for sore-throat relief. Special sections in each chapter explain the application of these herbs with children and pets too.
Over 25,000 copies in print.

Paper, 395 pages, $16.95, ISBN: 0-934252-48-3

• • •

DHEA: THE ULTIMATE REJUVENATING HORMONE
by Hasnain Walji, Ph.D.

A sane and balanced approach to the use of this age-slowing hormone, DHEA, which is fast being acknowledged as a new "wonder substance." Many studies indicate DHEA's positive usage for athletes and others concerned with losing weight without reducing caloric intake (DHEA blocks a fat-producing enzyme), as an aid to both short and long-term memory loss, and in such conditions as diabetes, cancer, Chronic Fatigue Syndrome, heart disease and immune system deficiencies. Contains a comprehensive but user-friendly review of research and relevant nutritional information.

Paper, 95 pages, $9. 95, ISBN: 0-934252-70-X

TO ORDER, PLEASE SEE ACCOMPANYING ORDER FORM.

ADDITIONAL TITLES OF INTEREST FROM HOHM PRESS

YOUR BODY CAN TALK: How to Listen to What Your Body Knows and Needs Through Simple Muscle Testing
by Susan L. Levy, D.C. and Carol Lehr, M.A.

Imagine having a diagnostic tool so sensitive that it could immediately tell you: • exactly how much protein...or fat...Your Body needs...• precisely which vitamins and minerals are needed in Your Diet...• what particular factors in the environment are depleting Your Vital Energy...• what hidden allergies you may have • which organs in your body are weakened due to over-stress • or anything else related to your health and well-being. You Already Have This Tool...at your own fingertips. Dr. Levy and Carol Lehr present clear instructions in *simple muscle testing*, together with over 25 simple tests for how to use it for specific problems or disease conditions. Special chapters deal with health problems specific to women (especially PMS and Menopause) and problems specific to men (like stress, heart disease, and prostate difficulties). Contains over 30 diagrams, plus a complete Index and Resource Guide.

Paper, 350 pages, $19.95, ISBN: 0-934252-68-8

• • •

NATURAL HEALING WITH HERBS
by Humbart "Smokey" Santillo, N.D.
Foreword by Robert S. Mendelsohn, M.D.

Dr. Santillo's first book, and Hohm Press' long-standing bestseller, is a classic handbook on herbal and naturopathic treatment. Acclaimed as the most comprehensive work of its kind, *Natural Healing With Herbs* details (in layperson's terms) the properties and uses of 120 of the most common herbs and lists comprehensive therapies for more than 140 common ailments. All in alphabetical order for quick reference.
Includes special sections on: • Diagnosis • How to make herbal remedies • The nature of health and disease • Diet and detoxification • Homeopathy... and more

Over 150,000 copies in print.
Paper, 408 pages, $16.95, ISBN: 0-934252-08-4

TO ORDER, PLEASE SEE ACCOMPANYING ORDER FORM.

ADDITIONAL TITLES OF INTEREST FROM HOHM PRESS

FOOD ENZYMES: THE MISSING LINK TO RADIANT HEALTH
by Humbart "Smokey" Santillo, N.D.

Immune system health is a subject of concern for everyone today. This book explains how the body's immune system, as well as every other human metabolic function, requires enzymes in order to work properly. Food enzyme supplementation is more essential today than ever before, since stress, unhealthy food, and environmental pollutants readily deplete them from the body. Humbart Santillo's breakthrough book presents the most current research in this field, and encourages simple, straightforward steps for how to make enzyme supplementation a natural addition to a nutrition-conscious lifestyle.
Special sections on: • Longevity and disease • The value of raw food and juicing • Detoxification • Prevention of allergies and candida • Sports and nutrition

Over 200,000 copies in print.
Paper, 108 pages, U.S. $7.95, ISBN: 0-934252-40-8 (English)

Now available in Spanish language version.
Paper, 108 pages, U.S. $6.95, ISBN: 0-934252-49-1 (Spanish)

■ Audio version of Food Enzymes
2 cassette tapes, 150 minutes, U.S. $17.95, ISBN: 0-934252-29-7

• • •

INTUITIVE EATING: EveryBody's Guide to Vibrant Health and Lifelong Vitality Through Food
by Humbart "Smokey" Santillo, N.D.

The natural voice of the body has been drowned out by the shouts of addictions, over-consumption, and devitalized and preserved foods. Millions battle the scale daily, experimenting with diets and nutritional programs, only to find their victories short-lived at best, confusing and demoralizing at worst. *Intuitive Eating* offers an alternative—a tested method for: • strengthening the immune system • natural weight loss • increasing energy • making the transition from a degenerative diet to a regenerative diet • slowing the aging process.

Paper, 450 pages, $16.95, ISBN: 0-934252-27-0

TO ORDER, PLEASE SEE ACCOMPANYING ORDER FORM.

ADDITIONAL TITLES OF INTEREST FROM HOHM PRESS

ARE YOU GETTING IT 5 TIMES A DAY?
Fruits and Vegetables
by Sydney H. Crackower, M.D., Barry A. Bohn, M.D. and
Rodney Langlinais, Reg. Pharmacist

The evidence is irrefutable. Research from around the world, and from
the American Cancer Society and the National Cancer Institute in the
U.S. agree ... 5 servings of nature's disease fighters—raw fruits and
vegetables—would markedly reduce cancer...stroke...and heart disease,
the leading killers of our times. Fresh fruits and vegetables, as well as an
intelligently pursued regimen of antioxidants, live enzymes and high fiber
are the nutritional basics of good health. This concise and straightforward
book will give you all the background research and practical steps you
need to start getting it today!

Paper, 78 pages, $ 6.95, ISBN: 0-934252-35-1

• • •

■ *HERBS, NUTRITION AND HEALING ;* AUDIO CASSETTE SERIES
by Dr. Humbart "Smokey" Santillo, N.D.

Santillo's most comprehensive seminar series. Topics covered in-depth
include: • the history of herbology • specific preparation of herbs for
tinctures, salves, concentrates, etc. • herbal dosages in both acute and
chronic illnesses • use of cleansing and transition diets • treating colds
and flu... and more.

4 cassettes, 330 minutes, $40.00, ISBN: 0-934252-22-X

• • •

■ *NATURE HEALS FROM WITHIN;* AUDIO CASSETTE SERIES
by Dr. Humbart "Smokey" Santillo, N.D.

How to take the next step in improving your life and health through
nutrition. Topics include: • The innate wisdom of the body. • The essential
role of elimination and detoxification • Improving digestion • How
"transition dieting" will take off the weight—for good! • The role of
heredity, diet, and prevention in health • How to overcome tiredness,
improve your immune system and live longer...and happier.

1 cassette, $8.95, ISBN: 0-934252-66-1

TO ORDER, PLEASE SEE ACCOMPANYING ORDER FORM.

ADDITIONAL TITLES OF INTEREST FROM HOHM PRESS

■ *LIVE SEMINAR ON FOOD ENZYMES*; AUDIO CASSETTE SERIES
by Dr. Humbart "Smokey" Santillo, N.D.

An in-depth discussion of the properties of food enzymes, describing their valuable use to maintain vitality, immunity, health and longevity. A must for anyone interested in optimal health. Complements all the information in the book.

1 cassette, $8.95, ISBN: 0-934252-29-7

• • •

■ *FRUITS AND VEGETABLES—The Basis of Health*; AUDIO CASSETTE SERIES
by Dr. Humbart "Smokey" Santillo, N.D.

Juicing of fruits and vegetables is one of the fastest and most efficient ways to supply the body with the raw food nutrients and enzymes needed to maintain optimal health. Explains the essential difference between a live food diet, which heals the body, and degenerative foods, which weaken the immune system and cause disease. Recipes included.

1 cassette, $8.95, ISBN: 0-934252-65-3

• • •

■ *WEIGHT-LOSS SEMINAR*; AUDIO CASSETTE SERIES
by Dr. Humbart "Smokey" Santillo, N.D.

"The healthiest people in the world know the secret of weight loss," says Santillo in this candid, practical, and information-based seminar. "If your body is getting what it needs, the appetite automatically turns off!" The reason for overweight is that we are starving ourselves to death, based on the improper balance of nutrients from our current food sources. This seminar explains the worthlessness of most dietary regimens and explodes many common myths about weight gain. Santillo stresses: • The essential distinction between "good" fats and "bad" fats • The necessity for protein and how to use it efficiently • How to get our primary vitamins and minerals from food • How to ease into becoming an "intuitive eater" so that the body is always getting what it knows it needs.

1 cassette, $8.95, ISBN: 0-934252-75-0

TO ORDER, PLEASE SEE ACCOMPANYING ORDER FORM

ADDITIONAL TITLES OF INTEREST FROM HOHM PRESS

10 ESSENTIAL FOODS
by Lalitha Thomas

Lalitha has done for food what she did with such wit and wisdom for herbs in her best-selling *10 Essential Herbs*. This new book presents 10 ordinary, but *essential* and great-tasting foods that can: • Strengthen a weakened immune system • Rebalance brain chemistry • Fight cancer and other degenerative diseases • Help you lose weight, simply and naturally.

Carrots, broccoli, almonds, grapefruit and six other miracle foods will enhance your health when used regularly and wisely. Lalitha gives in-depth nutritional information plus flamboyant and good-humored stories about these foods, based on her years of health and nutrition counseling. Each chapter contains easy and delicious recipes, tips for feeding kids and helpful hints for managing your food dollar. A bonus section supports the use of 10 Essential Snacks.

"This book's focus is squarely on target: fruits, vegetables and whole grains—everything comes in the right natural proportions."—Charles Attwood, M.D., F.A.A.P.; author, *Dr. Attwoods Low-Fat Prescription for Kids* (Viking).

Paper, 300 pages, $16.95, ISBN: 0-934252-74-2

• • •

THE MELATONIN AND AGING SOURCEBOOK
by Dr. Roman Rozencwaig, M.D. and Dr. Hasnain Walji, Ph.D.

"This is the most comprehensive reference on melatonin, yet published. It is an indispensable tool for those scientists, researchers, and physicians engaged in anti-aging therapeutics." —Dr. Ronald Klatz, President, American Academy of Anti-aging Medicing

This book covers the latest research on the pineal...control of aging, melatonin and sleep, melatonin and immunity, melatonin's role in cancer treatment, antioxidant qualities of melatonin, dosages, counter indications, quality control, and use with other drugs, melatonin application to heart disease, Alzheimer's, diabetes, stress, major depression, seasonal affective disorders, AIDS, SIDS, cataracts, autism...and many other conditions.

Cloth, 220 pages, $79.95, ISBN: 0-934252-73-4

TO ORDER, PLEASE SEE ACCOMPANYING ORDER FORM.

RETAIL ORDER FORM FOR HOHM PRESS HEALTH BOOKS

me_____ Phone (   ) _____

eet Address or P.O. Box _____

y _____State _____ Zip Code _____

QTY	TITLE	ITEM PRICE	TOTAL PRICE	
	10 ESSENTIAL FOODS	$16.95		
	10 ESSENTIAL HERBS	$16.95		
	ARE YOU GETTING IT 5 TIMES A DAY?	$6.95		
	DHEA: The Ultimate Rejuvenating Hormone	$9.95		
	FOOD ENZYMES/ENGLISH	$7.95		
	FOOD ENZYMES/SPANISH	$6.95		
	FOOD ENZYMES BOOK/AUDIO	$17.95		
	FRUITS & VEGETABLES/AUDIO	$8.95		
	HERBS, NUTRITION AND HEALING/AUDIO	$40.00		
	INTUITIVE EATING	$16.95		
	LIVE SEMINAR ON FOOD ENZYMES/AUDIO	$8.95		
	THE MELATONIN AND AGING SOURCEBOOK	$79.95		
	NATURAL HEALING WITH HERBS	$16.95		
	NATURE HEALS FROM WITHIN/AUDIO	$8.95		
	WEIGHT LOSS SEMINAR/AUDIO	$8.95		
	YOUR BODY CAN TALK: How to Listen...	$19.95		

RFACE SHIPPING CHARGES

ook $4.00

 additional item $1.00

SUBTOTAL:		
SHIPPING: (see below)		
TOTAL:		

P MY ORDER

☐ Surface U.S. Mail—Priority   ☐ UPS (Mail + $2.00)

☐ 2nd-Day Air (Mail + $5.00)   ☐ Next-Day Air (Mail + $15.00)

THOD OF PAYMENT:

☐ Check or M.O.   Payable to Hohm Press, P.O. Box 2501, Prescott, AZ 86302

☐ Call 1-800-381-2700 to place your credit card order

☐ Or call 1-520-717-1779 to fax your credit card order

☐ Information for Visa/MasterCard order only:

 #_____–_____–_____–_____ Expiration Date _____

ORDER NOW! Call 1-800-381-2700 or fax your order to 1-520-717-1779.
(Remember to include your credit card information.)